A TEST OF COURAGE.

Dedication

To my family with love. To Kevin, who is a staunch friend, and to Josh whose technical skill is unsurpassed.

A TEST OF COURAGE.

Chapter One

November in England. It was dark by 4.30pm, the shops were brightly lit and decorated for Christmas, and the aroma of roasting chestnuts hung fragrant in the chill air. Gabrielle remembered walking through the snow to midnight mass and listening to carol singers in the small village she had been born in.

She let go of the memories, staring out of the window at mile after mile of arid land, dotted with sheep and cows. Seven in the evening, judging by the shadows moving across the sunlit fields. The Australian November was unlike anything Gabrielle had ever experienced.

She had arrived in Australia two days previously, leaving England in the grip of an icy winter with all the attendant calamities, burst pipes, shortage of coal, and perilous trips into London to finalize her passport and flight arrangements.

Alighting in Darwin at 1.30am, she was stunned by the steam bath humidity as passengers for Sydney boarded another plane.

Unsuitably dressed in winter suit and long boots, she stared at the aircraft staff, men in shorts, with long socks and white shirts, and women in light summer uniforms. With little exception all tanned and healthy looking. She felt anaemic by comparison, too jet lagged to care.

The flight to Sydney was a blur, Gabrielle had been booked into a small hotel in the notorious King's Cross area, planning to continue her journey to South Australia by train after a decent night's sleep and a luxurious hot bath. Brushing her long blonde hair, she realised her summer wardrobe was woefully inadequate, and wondered if there were any inexpensive shops in the area.

The bath was heaven after the long hours of travel. She could not comprehend that she was in Australia to live, unlike the first trip some months previously.

She mused on the last weeks in England, remembering the wail of an ambulance, entering the Accident and Emergency Bay, only one of the sounds contributing to the hum of activity in the surgical ward office.

Gabrielle had turned her attention again to Hugh Evans, the urbane, grey suited man, standing by her desk. He'd smiled, acknowledging her momentary distraction.

"Always a place for you here if you tire of domesticity."

His gaze took in her blonde beauty, aware, she would be sorely missed. Her quiet common sense, good humour, and sheer hard work endeared her to colleagues, and patients alike.

Already, the female surgical ward was changing in response to the style of the newly appointed senior registered nurse. He hoped the ward would continue to run as smoothly as it had in the six years of Gabrielle's administration.

"It'll take at least a year to get used to marriage, and a different country, especially since Richard is intent on my input into the firm. "

Smiling, her gray eyes shone.

"From ward sister to legal secretary, I hope Richard appreciates your versatility."

She laughed. "Hugh, you're heavily biased in my favour, I shall miss that in the depths of South Australia."

She recalled Hugh's parting words, surprised by the quick hug when she left the farewell party several hours later. With much laughter, and calls of 'good luck, we'll miss you'.

She had been presented with a superb canteen of flatware, wedding and farewell gift combined.

Back in the present, refreshed by the bath and a snack in the hotel dining room, she spent several hours in the Cross, returning to the hotel without a purchase.

The following day she boarded the train, thankful that in a few hours she would reach her destination.

Now, still weary from her long plane journey, she watched the unfamiliar countryside slip past, lulled by the rhythmic sway of the carriage, anticipating with keen pleasure her reunion with her fiancé, Richard.

Her reverie was interrupted by the porter, announcing that the evening meal was being served in the restaurant car. She made her way along the corridor, and was seated at the table, studying the menu, when a cultured male voice asked.

"Pardon me, may I join you?"

Hesitating, she caught the eye of the waiter, who hastened to her side.

"We're short of tables, Ma'am, if you could share?"

She smiled and nodded, as the tall, impeccably dressed man seated himself opposite, extending his hand.

"Connor Quinlan, forgive the interruption."

She was quietly pleased at the prospect of companionship, and said so, adding,

"Good cuisine is always enhanced by pleasant company, hallo, I'm Gabrielle Graham, 'though not for long."

Encouraged by his quizzical expression, she explained.

"I'm getting married in a fortnight."

Quinlan beckoned the waiter.

"In that case, we must celebrate with champagne."

Several glasses later, and chatting more in the manner of friends than casual acquaintances, Gabrielle wondered aloud why it seemed easier to share confidences with total strangers.

"Perhaps, because we're ships in the night?"

Connor offered, with an enigmatic smile.

She acknowledged that. "It's as well, seeing I've bored you with my life history."

Talking, they watched, as the huge orange sun sank beneath the skyline, and the train crossed the border into South Australia.

She slept soundly that night, a combination of exhaustion, and champagne. At breakfast the next morning, she was seated, when Quinlan appeared; beckoning to him, she indicated the seat opposite.

In full daylight, she realised he was startlingly handsome, thick black hair and blue green eyes, his powerful build made more apparent in the tailored suit.

She admitted to herself that he would be alarmingly easy to fall for. Handsome,cultured, easy to confide in, compassionate.

Compared with Richard…..no, why would she even begin to compare the two? Uneasy at the thought, she gave her full attention to Connor.

As she listened to Connor describing his work as a volunteer at a women's refuge, she thought. 'Richard would never do that', and "why can't I rely on Richard for that?' disliking the thought that she was critical of her fiancé, however true the thought.

The morning passed quickly in Quinlan's company, and it was with a sense of regret that Gabrielle said farewell to him that afternoon. Apart from Quinlan's good looks, he gave the impression of genuine warmth, and his wicked sense of humour was irresistible.

The train was on time arriving in Adelaide, and Gabrielle disembarked, gazing along the platform, heart thumping at the thought of Richard's imminent arrival. As passengers left the station, she checked her watch, Richard, usually so punctual, was conspicuously late.

Fifteen minutes became thirty, and she sought a telephone booth, dialing Richard's home number, and listening to his recorded message. He would surely be here soon. She returned to the dingy waiting room to wash her hands and apply fresh lipstick.

On the platform outside, travelers streamed from the train which had stopped shortly before. She realised with shock that almost an hour had passed and still no sign of Richard.

Quickly, she found a porter, and boarded a taxi, waiting until her luggage was stowed in the boot. The only activity when the taxi stopped outside the elegant two-story house thirty minutes later was the grey, brown wattlebird perched in a flowering gum.

"You want the cases out, Miss?"

She forced a tremulous smile, tired and dispirited she was at a loss to understand Richard's absence.

"Thanks, I have a key, I'd appreciate it if you would bring my suitcases in."

The hall was cold and untidy, boxes and newspapers scattered randomly. She stared, shivering involuntarily.

Behind her, the taxi driver whistled.

"Not much of a welcome, Miss."

Perplexed, she walked through the rooms, thankful for the man's presence.

"I don't understand, my fiancé knew I was arriving tonight."

The man's face was noncommittal.

"There's a decent hotel in town, you'll get a hot meal and a room for the night. It will give you time to sort something out tomorrow."

He placed a tentative hand on her shoulder, aware of her distress.

" Shall I take your cases to the car? It'll only take five minutes to get to the Grove Hotel."

She nodded, close to tears, stumbling after him as he reloaded the luggage, and closed the front door. As Ian Kaye promised, the Grove hotel was warm and inviting. Her cases were deposited at reception, and Ian bade her goodbye, adding.

"Good luck Miss, this is the cab company's phone number if you need transport tomorrow."

She thanked him, accepting the card.

After a light meal, she showered and lay on the bed, tired, but too overwrought to sleep. Television offered a quiz show, football, and a James Bond rerun, with Connery foiling villains and rescuing the beautiful heroine. Soothed by the improbable plot, she slept.

It was a glorious day. From her viewpoint atop the cliffs, Gabrielle gazed at the undulant country, green and fertile. In a cloudless blue sky a kestrel circled, dropping to snare some unseen prey.

Startled by the sound of Richard's voice, she turned, smiling as he sat beside her running his hand through unruly dark hair. Curiously, his bulk seemed insubstantial. She reached out to touch him, reassuring herself of his presence, at the instant he slipped, panic etched on his face, and fell over the edge of the precipice.

Horror struck; she knelt looking down to where Richard's still body lay on the rocks below. A single piercing scream woke her to the cool stillness of the hotel room. A nightmare, little wonder given her anxiety at Richard's unexplained absence.

Her travel clock showed the time to be 6.15am, too early for hotel staff to have the dining room open. The small well-stocked fridge contained a carton of milk and a sealed pack of Earl Grey tea.

In minutes, she returned to bed, turning on both bedside lights and rummaging in her hold all, for pen and notepad. Sipping her tea, she thought of the events preceding her departure from England.

Richard had phoned the night before her journey, she'd presumed from the house, although now she was unsure. On reflection, she realised with a sense of relief that Richard's domestic, May Burns, might know where he was.

She had met May on one occasion in July, when she stayed with Richard after their engagement was announced. She recalled how comfortable she felt with the practical, sturdily built woman, whose calm presence brought order to Richard's often chaotic pace.

Chapter Two

She pictured Connor Quinlan, toasting her with champagne, she hoped he was faring better than she.

May Burns would be easy to locate, Richard had no family, and the law firm at which he was a partner would provide an idea of his whereabouts.

Reassured, she climbed out of bed and walked across to the window. Already, the rising sun painted the sky with pink fingers.

Below in the street a muscular young man lifted a dustbin with ease, depositing the contents into the slowly moving garbage truck. She was comforted by the ordinary scene; she had been a continent away when last she saw a garbage truck. Traffic was building in the street below, and more pedestrians appeared.

Out in the hall the lift doors opened and closed, and the quiet hum of conversation, punctuated by laughter, could be heard. She showered, anticipating breakfast and dressing in a cool linen suit and low-heeled shoes, neat and functional.

At 8.15am, she phoned the number Ian Kaye had given her and asked for a taxi at 9am. In the dining room, the aroma of coffee, and bacon made her aware of her hunger.

She was shown to a table laid for one, and ordered cereal, toast, marmalade, and fruit juice, reflecting that lunch might be hours away depending on what the morning brought.

The taxi arrived promptly at 9am. She gave an address to the driver, disappointed not to see Ian Kaye. By day the town appeared larger and busier than she remembered from the previous visit.

Outside Richard's house she asked the driver to wait, expecting Richard to have returned from wherever he had been. She was at a loss to understand why he hadn't left her a message.

She was prepared to keep an open mind however, in the event of his continued absence, trusting that whatever had delayed him would be explained. Immediately she opened the door it was apparent the house was unoccupied. Returning to the taxi she paid the driver, carrying her hand luggage to the veranda whilst he dealt with the larger cases.

Inside, the cool quiet atmosphere was unchanged. Again she walked through the rooms, ascending the staircase to check the upper floor.

In the master bedroom where she had stayed with Richard a few short months previously, nothing had changed, although she noted a fine layer of dust covering the furniture.

She frowned, May Burns had seemed competent, the house immaculate on her first visit, months before.

Retracing her steps she looked for an envelope, a note, a clue to Richard's whereabouts. Finding nothing, she rang the Pearce and Raglan firm of lawyers, his workplace.

'Pearce and Raglan, how may I help you?'

Cheryl, the receptionist Gabrielle had met once, acknowledged her, then placed the call on hold, explaining any calls regarding Mr. Pearce were to be put through to Mr. Raglan.

"Gabrielle, thank the Lord. I've been trying to contact you, where are you, do you have transport?"

Momentarily shaken, she replied, "I'm at the house, I don't have a car."

" No problem, I'll be there soon."

Concerned before, now serious doubt surfaced, she looked around the room, completely at a loss to understand what was happening.

Had Richard been involved in an accident, if so, why hadn't someone phoned her?

Numerous questions flooded her mind. She heard a car pull up and jumped to her feet. From the window she saw Daniel's Volvo in the driveway.

Daniel's face betrayed nothing as he greeted her, asking her when she had arrived. She explained, adding how surprised and then anxious she became at Richard's absence.

Daniel's face was grim, looking at the disordered hall he asked.

"Any milk in the fridge, I could do with a coffee?"

She apologized. "I'm so bewildered I've forgotten the most basic courtesy."

Daniel followed her into the kitchen, moving to the fridge to check its contents, while she collected coffee and mugs.

"Yes, there's milk, but it's curdled."

He held the carton away from him.

"I'll tip this in the garden otherwise it'll make the kitchen smell."

She filled the kettle, spooning coffee into mugs, and, on Daniel's return, asked.

"Is Decaf all right, there's nothing else?"

He sat at the table watching her with an unreadable expression on his face while seconds passed without a word exchanged. She carried both mugs and the sugar bowl to the table.

"Daniel, if you've any idea what's happening please tell me."

Slowly, choosing his words with care, he asked.

"When did you last see Richard?"

She frowned. "You know that, July, six months ago when I applied for registration."

Nodding, he confirmed. "You came to the office I remember".

Perplexed, she stared at him. Raglan, not a handsome man, could be described as rugged. Tall and broad shouldered, with curly brown hair, and hazel eyes, he possessed a sharp intellect. He reached out to take her hand,

"Gabrielle, there's no easy way to tell you, so I'll just say it, Richard's been embezzling money from the firm. The accountants don't have an exact figure yet, but it's well over two million."

She gasped, blood draining from her face; Daniel rose, rounding the table to place both hands on her shoulders.

"I realise it's pointless to tell you not to worry, it's an alarming situation."

Dazed, she asked, "did no one suspect something was amiss?"

He resumed his seat. "Drink your coffee, you're white as a sheet".

In a quieter tone he continued. "Richard had control of the trust accounts, Pearce Raglan have some very wealthy clients, he's been diverting funds to a private bank account for Lord knows how long."

She stared at him. "He sounded as he usually did when I spoke to him on Friday evening. He said he couldn't wait for me to get here."

Daniel pushed his mug away. "I've known Richard for years, we were at Uni together, I always thought he was... different, I suppose. What you saw wasn't always what you got. You know as much as I do. All I can say is we must stay focused."

He grimaced at his own words.

"Does anyone else in the firm know?"

"Obviously both accountants, and Malcolm."

(Daniel's father, and a senior partner in the firm.)

She was thankful for Daniel's calm unruffled acceptance of what was for him, an unmitigated disaster.

She knew nothing of the law firm's clients. However it wasn't difficult to imagine the damage this kind of fraud would do to the practice Malcolm and Daniel had painstakingly built over a dozen years.

Glancing at his watch, Daniel stood up.

"I must go, are you staying here for the time being?"

"I haven't given it any thought; I suppose if Richard wants to contact me it will be here."

Daniel agreed." Gabrielle, meet me tonight at the Grove Hotel, say 7pm."

He took her hand, his brown eyes serious,

"Stay calm, we'll get through this somehow."

She managed a smile, 'I'll see you tonight, if Richard phones before that I'll contact you."

The house seemed deserted after he left.

Chapter Three

She was dazed by his revelation of Richard's deceit. She returned to the kitchen, looking through the dresser drawers for a notepad. Her mind raced, she saw Richard's face, heard the excitement in his voice. She had attributed it to his joy that she would soon be with him.

Or was he excited about the money, safely deposited in a bank account somewhere; of the freedom it would bring to continue the lifestyle he was accustomed to.

He schemed, while she made final preparations to join him in Australia. Keep busy, her inner voice told her, don't think about Richard. The wedding... ten days from now. The wedding had been planned when she had visited months before.

She must phone her parents. Tears ran unchecked down her face at the thought of their bewilderment.

She would phone this evening; she did not want to alarm them more than was inevitable by crying when she told them of Richard's defection.

She reheated the coffee and poured a generous splash of whisky into the mug. What did it matter if she was unsteady on her feet? Her hands were shaky, she was bereft, shocked.

Usually abstinent, the alcohol blunted her feelings of despair, she was a mature responsible adult, she would survive.

Staying in the house meant shopping, checking fuel for the Aga, letting the neighbours know she was occupying the house. Apart from the lack of milk, Richard had a plentiful supply of groceries.

There were logs in the shed outside, and, in the freezer, neatly packaged and labelled containers of meat, fish, and vegetables. She lit the woodstove, grateful for the warmth which gradually spread through the kitchen.

She was cold despite the sunny day. The treachery of Richard's behaviour astounded her, she stared at the diamond ring on her finger, it meant little now.

She recalled Richard showing her the wood stove. It heated water he said, which was piped around the house via radiators in all the rooms.

He had taken her through the house, too large for one, (he kissed her on the cheek), but perfect for both. Despite her misgivings she would give him the benefit of the doubt. Outside, the garage door was locked and she wondered where the key was kept.

In the kitchen, she looked around all the likely places, finding six or more unmarked keys in a covered dish on the dresser.

The third key she tried unlocked the garage door and the small shed she had peered into the window of when she sought fuel for the Aga.

Assuming Richard had taken his car, she was stunned to see the Jaguar in its usual place. By now she was ceasing to question Richard's behaviour, thankful to have the car at her disposal.

Coming out of the garage, she noticed an attractive middle aged woman hanging clothes on the line in the garden next door.

 She hoped the woman wouldn't notice her reddened eyes or hear the tremble in her voice.

Smiling, the woman introduced herself. "We thought Richard was back?"

"No, I'm Gabrielle Graham, Richard's fiancée, I'm staying here until he returns."

"Nothing wrong I hope, we wondered when he would be back, it's not like him to go without asking us to keep an eye on the house."

She agreed, saying, "Oh what a tangled web we weave. "

"When first we practice to deceive?"

Startled, she looked up into Connor Quinlan's smiling eyes, feeling her heart miss a beat.

"The bride to be and fiancé I presume?"

She gathered her wits. "Connor, what a surprise, this is Daniel Raglan, Richard's law partner."

The men shook hands, Daniel's manner stiff and formal.

Eyebrows raised, Quinlan asked, "Raglan, as in Pearce Raglan?"

"The same."

Daniel's terse reply bordered on rudeness.

She flashed Quinlan a dazzling smile in unspoken apology for Daniel's hostility, wondering why he was in Adelaide.

"Care to join us for a pre-dinner drink?"

"Regrettably, I must take a rain check, I'm meeting a colleague." Smiling down at her, he took her hand, exerting a slight pressure.

" Perhaps I could phone you? "

She took the pen Daniel offered and wrote Quinlan's phone number on a serviette.

"Connor, am I late?"

She stared at the newcomer ; if Quinlan was handsome this woman was stunning. Only inches shorter than Quinlan, she was slender, yet full breasted.

The black hair, in a classic chignon, contrasted sharply with heavily lashed, sapphire eyes, her cool smile revealed perfect teeth.

"Olivia, this is Gabrielle Graham, and Daniel Raglan."

Quinlan looked at her, gauging her reaction to the newcomer. Gabrielle, aware she was staring, turned to Daniel amused to see that he too, was staring at this incredibly beautiful woman.

Taking Quinlan's arm, Olivia urged. "We must go, we'll miss the overture."

Quinlan shrugged." No rush. Gabrielle, I'll be in touch, nice to meet you, Raglan."

A smile at Gabrielle, and he was gone. She recovered first, teasing Daniel, who still gazed after Olivia. "Gorgeous, isn't she?"

"Awesome, women like that make me nervous. So you met Quinlan on the train?"

Gabrielle nodded, "I didn't expect to see him again although he did say he worked in the city."

"What does he do? He looks like a professional, a lawyer or doctor, he's no blue collar worker...."

Gabrielle shook her head. "Daniel I've no idea, what does it matter?"

Finishing their drinks, they walked to the restaurant. During dinner, the implications of Richard's embezzlement occupied the conversation, and it was after 11pm when they left the restaurant.

She was thankful she had the Jaguar at her disposal, refusing Daniel's offer to follow her to the house and promising to keep in touch.

Garaging the car, she walked through the kitchen, deciding against a hot drink. The wood stove took seconds to bank for the night, and leaving the hall light on she walked upstairs to the master bedroom.

Her last thought before sleep overtook her was to wonder about the relationship between Quinlan and Olivia. There was a commitment of some kind, judging by Olivia's proprietary behaviour towards him.

She was up and showered early next morning, intent on looking at the contents of the roll top desk, and then phoning the local hospital to inquire about a job.

Staying in Adelaide would give her the opportunity to learn something about Richard's whereabouts hopefully. She put a c.d. of Vivaldi in the tape deck as she tried various keys, not surprised that none fitted. She was loathe to use force on the beautiful old desk.

Looking through the Rolodex on Richard's desk she located May Burn's telephone number, dialing and listening to the tone.

May probably had other cleaning jobs and would be home this evening. A brief call to Daniel who had no news, however she was happy to learn that the Q.E.H was one of the biggest hospitals to apply for work. Daniel had obliged to research hospitals in the area.

Chapter Four

She heard a raised voice, then laughter, thinking that perhaps mail had been delivered to the neighbours. Opening the front door, she smiled at the startled postman, introducing herself as Richard's fiancée.

" I haven't seen Mr. Pearce for a couple of weeks, his mail's being held at the Post Office in Adelaide. If you sign a statuary declaration you should be able to collect it for him."

She was beginning to realise Richard's disappearance had been well planned, how ironic that she anticipated their future as he forsook his former life.

Returning to the lounge she phoned the Q.E.H, arranging to meet the nursing administrator that afternoon to explore job possibilities.

At a loss to occupy herself, she washed her breakfast dishes.

The dishwasher was more suited to a large family, or washing dishes after entertaining dinner guests, one of Richard's favourite ways to spend an evening, a catered dinner for friends and colleagues.

She checked her watch then dialed May's number, gratified to hear May's familiar voice.

May's concern was apparent, Mr. Pearce had given her a month's notice she said, suddenly and with no apparent reason. He had written a glowing reference, certainly her work was not at fault.

Gabrielle mentioned her appointment at the Queen Elizabeth hospital, asking if May would be at home in the next fifteen minutes.

The house was not far from the hospital, and soon she was being welcomed into the small immaculate house.

May greeted her, taking her hand. "A troubling start, to your first week in a new country."

She led her into the kitchen, apologizing.

"I'm icing my grand daughter's birthday cake; will you have a cup of coffee while I finish it?"

Gabrielle accepted, eager to hear May's account of her dismissal, watching as the cake was decorated and trimmed with tiny candles. Gabrielle asked May what had happened in the few days before Richard disappeared.

"Mr. Pearce changed in the last few months I looked after him, he wasn't the man I started working for a few years back".

She frowned. "He was usually so easy going. Always a smile and a joke. Then he started drinking, several times he was in bed when I arrived for work, and there were liquor bottles in the lounge and kitchen, the house smelt of it."

The look she gave Gabrielle was compassionate.

"Sorry dear, no point beating around the bush; he became so irritable I thought I'd be better off giving him my notice. I came in one day when he was talking on the 'phone, he glared at me and waved me away."

" I could see he was upset. He rarely smoked in the house before, and then he started getting through several packs a week, ash everywhere and the house reeking".

Glancing at her May said, "I thought he was in some kind of trouble, but it wasn't my business to say anything. Finally, he called me at home and said he didn't need me to clean for him anymore, he'd send a cheque and a reference."

Wiping her hands on a tea towel, she added. "That was the last I heard 'til you arrived."

Gabrielle gazed into the fire, disappointed, but knowing only Richard had all the answers.

"Our wedding is twelve days away and I've no idea where he is or if he'll be back. I hoped you'd know something. Anything... "

She stood, gathering her coat and bag. "Thank you for the coffee, I'm sorry to have troubled you."

May opened the front door." No worries, if you hear anything please phone me, I do hope he contacts you soon."

'Little chance of that', Gabrielle thought. May would be shocked at Richard's duplicity had she known the reason for his behaviour. She reached the Q.E.H. well before her appointment, using the time to locate the nursing admin: office. Standing before the bank of lifts her thoughts were interrupted by a light touch on her shoulder.

"We must stop meeting like this."

Connor's smile was teasing. Gabrielle's heart leaped. Laughing, she nodded.

"You appear when I least expect it. Are you visiting someone?"

"I could say the same, 'though I would add, it's a pleasure to see you, and, no, I work here."

"Really, may I ask in what capacity? Oh, I need the second floor for nursing admin."

"Would it be presumptuous to ask why you want admin?"

She explained adding, "not full time, two or three shifts to start with until I have a clearer picture of what's happening."

Quinlan's face was noncommittal. "I see, and to answer your question I'm a clinical psychologist."

"My office is on the second floor along the corridor. Will you let me know how the interview goes?"

She laughed, aware that she was blushing. "Certainly. Forgive me, I'm rambling, probably nervous about the interview."

No need to tell him that her heart was pounding at his closeness. She had forgotten about the interview, so overwhelmed was she by his presence.

The interview went well, and she was assured a place would be found for her, part time initially and perhaps full time later if she wished.

"Experienced nursing sisters are worth their weight in gold," the Director of Nursing assured her.

Walking along the corridor she found Quinlan's office, entering when his voice responded to her knock.

"Miss Graham, and judging from your smile soon to be a staff member?"

"Connor, you didn't mention you worked at the Q.E.H, I hope I didn't disclose too many secrets on the train."

"I don't imagine you'd have secrets, or have I misjudged you?"

Aware of his eyes fixed on her face she smiled.

"Perhaps I should call you Doctor Quinlan, you're the mysterious one, you gave no indication on the train journey that you're a clinical psychologist."

"I didn't think it was relevant, and I promised your confidences would be respected although nothing you told me was R rated.

How are the wedding preparations coming along?"

She studied him, whilst he maintained silence aware of her inner turmoil.

"I haven't seen Richard since July; he wasn't at the station or at home when I arrived."

Surprised, Quinlan asked. "No note or message left for you?"

She shook her head, "I know why he left, it will soon be public knowledge."

Quinlan leaned forward on the desk, studying her face.

"Before you say anything let me tell you I'll help in any way I can, obviously whatever you tell me is confidential."

"Thank you; apart from Daniel I've no one to talk to.... "

Faltering, she briefly outlined what she knew, adding, "Daniel says the amount embezzled is conservatively around two million dollars.'

Quinlan whistled. "No wonder he took off, that's a fortune when it belongs to other people."

She agreed. "At this stage I would say the wedding is postponed, 'though I feel miserable about condemning Richard without giving him the chance to tell me why he's jeopardised everything."

Quinlan checked his diary.

"No more appointments, it's too soon to dine, and too late for lunch. Will you settle for cappuccino now and dinner later, or am I being presumptuous?"

Smiling, she agreed, her usual composure absent. He made her feel like a teenager in love for the first time.

Taking her arm he led her along the corridor, telling his secretary to page him only in the direst emergency.

Over coffee she finished telling what little she knew of Richard's disappearance. Quinlan was a good listener, his entire attention focused on her. They sat quietly after she finished speaking, then Quinlan asked, "What will you do about the wedding, have you told your family?"

"Not yet, I hoped Richard would contact me. Luckily it's only my immediate family, no friends or work colleagues which is a blessing."

Quinlan placed a gentle hand over hers.

"Well for better or worse, you're not on your own with this. I'll make a couple of phone calls then I'm entirely at your command."

Gabrielle smiled, comforted, as he wrote her phone number on a pad.

"My most pressing priority is to leave this house, and phone my family before they arrive for the wedding."

Standing, Quinlan towered over her, she felt secure, protected; fleetingly she hoped his partner realised how fortunate she was to have a man of Quinlan's integrity.

Her immediate impulse on entering the quiet house was to play the taped messages indicated by the glowing light. The first call was from Daniel. 'Was she free for dinner?'

 Then May Burns asking if she had news of Richard, and the now familiar female voice.

'Richard, please phone, Mum was here yesterday, I couldn't tell her where you were, I'm really concerned, how's Alex? '

'Mum? Alex?'

Chapter Five

She had no recollection of Richard mentioning his mother other than to tell her that his parents were dead, and who was Alex?

Daniel answered the office phone, he had no news concerning Richard, enquiring if she had plans for the evening. She asked for a rain check pleading a prior commitment, and not mentioning Quinlan.

She was aware Daniel preferred not to talk about Richard on the phone in case the conversation was overheard.

The doorbell chime startled her, if it was Quinlan she wasn't expecting him so early.

Six foot plus of masculine charm leaned against the door frame. He grinned, offering a bunch of freesias when she opened the door.

"I couldn't resist, I trust I'm not intruding?"

She welcomed him, expressing surprise.

"How did you know where the house was?"

"Easy, I looked for Pearce in the phone book."

Laughing, he admitted, "I knocked at three other doors before this one."

Arranging the fragrant blooms in a vase, she asked.

"Will you have a cup of coffee, or something stronger?"

"Coffee's fine."

He followed her into the kitchen, looking around.

"Your fiancé has expensive taste."

"Without the finances to indulge it, I waver between anger and a deep concern about him."

She busied herself preparing coffee.

"Natural enough." Quinlan accepted a mug. "I confess I'm curious from a professional and personal viewpoint.

"Professional? "

"Certainly, why a seemingly successful lawyer, a partner in a thriving practice with a beautiful fiancée and a good income, would destroy his credibility by embezzlement?"

"I didn't know him, obviously."

She curled a strand of blonde hair around her finger.

"I assumed he wanted marriage and eventually a family. He enjoyed my family, he said how lucky I was, his parents were dead, and he had no one."

Without hesitation, she told him of the phone call from a family member. "I can't even trace where the call's from."

Quinlan's face was sombre.

"Unfinished business, not knowing why he did what he did must be a huge frustration."

"My dreams lately, one dream in particular, where Richard falls over a cliff, and I can't get to him, scare me."

She looked at Quinlan.

"I've been off course since I left England. I'm used to being self-sufficient and knowing where I was going. The last few years have been secure and predictable, apart from the usual work hassles."

" Now I don't seem to have a grip on my life."

Pausing, she made eye contact with him.

"Sorry, I keep thinking this is a nightmare I'll wake up from, and Richard will be here."

"Don't apologise for something that's entirely messed up your life, I don't know any woman who, in your situation, would remain calm and cheerful."

She smiled, comforted by his observation, then recalling Richard's mail, reached for her carry all.

"I collected his letters, nothing significant with one exception."

She handed the envelope to` him. He examined the postmark, turning the letter over.

"No return address, are you going to open it?"

"Should I?"

Without waiting for his reply, she opened the envelope.

"From Jay, at least, that's the signature."

Silently she read it, unaware of Quinlan's steady gaze.

"Mm, Jay writes, 'Richard, why haven't you returned my calls, I must talk to you.'

No address, just the date."

She put the letter aside. Jay…. wondering what was Jay's connection with Richard?

"I spoke to my mother earlier, telling her the wedding has been 'delayed." Earlier, buoyed by the alcohol she consumed; she had phoned her parents knowing they were preparing for the journey.

She pictured her mother in the rambling old Tudor house, heard again the concern in her voice.

'Come home, as short or long a stay as you wish, your father is worried, we can't imagine Richard stealing from the firm, he certainly fooled us.'

She promised to write, whatever her fiancé's shortcomings, she was entirely blessed with her family.

Quinlan, looking surprisingly at home in the leather recliner, raised his dark eyebrows enquiringly as she sat opposite.

"All's well at home?"

She nodded, "I have a great family, loving, supportive, I've been spoiled, I suppose."

"You, spoilt…"

Quinlan's teeth flashed in a wide smile, and she laughed with him.

"Me. I don't mean material things, more freedom from family problems; no divorces, or disagreements, an occasional difference of opinion, which is respected, and always, love and support."

A comfortable silence, as the last notes of Schubert's 'Unfinished Symphony' faded. Quinlan indicated the C.D player.

"I didn't think you'd mind, there's a marvellous selection."

"I'm a classical music and blues fan, the Peggy Lee, Sarah Vaughn, and Miles Davis are mine."

Quinlan murmured his approval.

"Tell me if I overstep boundaries; do you co own the house?"

"No, Richard bought the house about the same time I became senior surgical R/n at Price General, 'though I didn't know him then."

"Mind if I ask who handles Richard's estate, who his executor is?"

She shrugged. "It wasn't something I asked, I expect Daniel would know; I never thought about Richard's wealth, I was so naïve, and far too trusting."

The grandfather clock in the hall struck the hour, Quinlan glanced at his watch.

"I've made a 'to be confirmed' booking at the Grove, are you up to it?"

"It's so peaceful here, would you mind if I said no?"

"Takeaway, then?"

"Chinese, and I promise not to mention Richard."

Quinlan laughed.

"Done, will you phone or shall I?"

Within the hour they were seated comfortably by the open fire, they had enjoyed their meal, eaten in the opulent dining room. Quinlan was an entertaining companion, seeming intent on diverting her thoughts from her absent fiancé.

He encouraged her curiosity about his life, she learned he was the only child of academic parents, whom he visited several times a year.

He consulted at the Q.E.H and had a private practice in the town. He spoke of his marriage whilst an undergraduate.

"Clare was taking a degree in anaesthesiology; shortly after our first anniversary, she was diagnosed with a kidney tumour, she died eight months later, despite chemo and radiotherapy."

She sat motionless, aware of his pain and unsure how to express her compassion.

Gazing into the distance, Quinlan concluded.

"After the funeral, the house was sold. I couldn't face living there with everything we chose together, using the wedding presents, seeing the herbs and shrubs she planted flourishing."

With obvious effort, his gaze became focused, looking across at her he remarked.

"Enough gloom for one evening, I wouldn't say no to a whisky, if you'll join me?"

"Please, the bar's in the library, I'll show you where."

Leaving him to mix drinks, she filled the ice bucket and returned to the sitting room. Quinlan handed her a cut glass tumbler, a look of enquiry on his face.

"I like an occasional malt, what I am addicted to, 'though, is my pipe."

"By all means".

She indicated an ashtray.

"I don't smoke, Richard did, and I much prefer to see a man smoke a pipe than a cigarette."

She enjoyed watching Quinlan fill the briar with tobacco, tamp and light it, sending puffs of aromatic smoke into the atmosphere.

"Very domesticated."

He flashed a devilish grin at her.

"Fine whisky, a good pipe, and a log fire, what more could I ask?"

He raised an eyebrow, his eyes speculative.

To her chagrin, a blush swept over her face; Quinlan's virile masculinity was impossible to ignore, more so if he chose to exert it, which he did now.

Contemplating her, his voice soft, he said.

"Pearce is a bloody fool, you're worth more than all the money he's taken."

"Pearce?"

It took a moment to comprehend his contemptuous use of Richard's surname. The space between them was electric. Putting the pipe down, he leaned forward taking both her hands in his.

"Gabrielle."

With no recollection of how it happened, she was in his arms, his lips burning on hers, the length of his muscular body pressed insistently against hers.

His mouth tasted of whisky, and curiously, peppermint. Murmuring, he cupped her head, fingers tangled in her curls as she melted into him.

The phone rang, shockingly loud in the quiet room.

She placed her hands against Quinlan's chest struggling to break away, almost falling as he released her, an unfathomable expression on his face.

Senses reeling, she picked up the phone, hearing Daniel's voice.

"Gabrielle, I've a paper trail, that'll give us some idea of Richard's whereabouts; it would appear he's in the States, Gabrielle?"

She hoped her voice was composed, aware of Quinlan lowering the volume on the C.D. player.

"The States?"

"As in the U.S.A; are you alright, you sound flustered?"

"America, why would he go to America?"

"Indeed, who's to know what his plans are, speaking of which, can we meet for lunch tomorrow?"

Arranging time and venue, she replaced the receiver, and walked back to the ottoman.

Quinlan had resumed his seat in the recliner, watching her with a quizzical expression. The pipe lay unheeded in the ashtray.

"Richard's in America, it seems we won't get married as arranged."

Quinlan reached for the pipe.

"You would have deep reservations about him now, he's done you a favour."

"I don't think he intended to get married."

Sitting opposite him, she felt completely relaxed, Richard had solved her dilemma by fleeing to America, taking matters out of her hands.

"It will take me a while to absorb the knowledge that Richard and I aren't fated to be together."

"No longer engaged?"

Quinlan's eyes searched her face.

She held his gaze steadfastly.

"Until I can speak to him, I consider the engagement over, although I feel as if I'm deserting a sinking ship."

"That presumes Richard will return, to accept responsibility for what he's done, do you think that's likely? "I've ceased trying to understand his behaviour, what I do feel is confusion, and a sense of abandonment."

Quinlan's expression was thoughtful.

"Indeed, you would."

With a pang, she remembered his loss. Quietly, aware of her expression, he said.

"I'll always love Clare. Thankfully, over time, I've come to terms with her death, and somehow, moved on. If anyone had told me that several years ago, I would have ignored them."

Leaning towards him, she placed her hand on his arm.

"Forgive me, I didn't mean to stir up memories for you."

His hand covered hers.

"Time I left, remember, I'm here if you need someone to talk to, I'll phone you tomorrow, perhaps we can catch up in the afternoon?"

"Yes, I'm meeting Daniel for lunch, then I plan on going to the hospital, to get a feel for the place."

Quinlan brushed her cheek with his lips. "Talk to you tomorrow."

Chapter Six

She slept well that night, free of the troubling dream of Richard falling. Despite the late night, she felt relaxed and optimistic the next morning, eager for the day ahead. The forecast was for sunshine and a mild day.

She was surprised at her reflection in the mirror; she had lost weight, making her eyes look huge, a perfect foil for her blonde hair.

She knew the aqua trouser suit accentuated her curves, and chose her shoes carefully, they must be comfortable for walking. She wondered if Quinlan was at the hospital today, feeling a shiver of anticipation at the thought of seeing him.

Checking the pantry, she made a shopping list. Richard, or rather, May Burns, had stocked the shelves fully with different ingredients from which a variety of meals could be made, with the addition of vegetables, and a knowledge of cooking.

Again, she was glad the freezer was stacked with poultry, meat, and seafood.

She thought it was sufficient to last one person for months, particularly since Richard had shown a marked preference for dining out in the few months she had known him.

She wondered if Quinlan, despite his sophisticated persona, enjoyed home cooking.

She was a talented cook, wanting to share her gift with someone who appreciated it, so much more fun than cooking for one.

Over lunch Daniel repeated his news, adding that a private investigator had traced Richard to New York.

"He used travelers' cheques and made several purchases with a visa, so it wasn't difficult for the P. I."

Wiping his lips, he beckoned a waiter.

"Two cappuccinos."

When the young man left, Daniel asked.

"How are you holding up? I must say, you look gorgeous."

"Oddly, knowing Richard's in America has liberated me, I'm not waiting for the other shoe to drop".

The cappuccinos were placed in front of them. Smiling her thanks at the waiter, she took a sip, gazing at Daniel over the rim of the cup.

"I'm looking forward to starting at the Q.E.H, I'd like to stay in the house, until I find accommodation unless that causes problems?"

"Richard owns the house; at the moment the firm has no plans to repossess through litigation, the same with the house contents and the Jaguar. "

"We want the money he embezzled since he bought the house, although if that isn't an option, Malcolm wants all Richard's assets seized."

She winced, then shrugging, asked.

"What are your plans?"

"I'm bound for New York to see if something can be salvaged from this mess. Neither Malcolm nor I want adverse publicity, so there'll be no witch hunt."

Surprised, she asked. "You know where Richard is?"

'At present; if he moves he'll be traced."

"When do you leave for America?"

"Tomorrow, do you want me to give him a message?"

Her eyes flashed.

"What I have to say to him must be said face to face."

"Fair enough, and now I must make tracks, have you seen anything of Quinlan by the way?"

She blushed, avoiding his scrutiny.

"Well that answers my question."

"Not really, he has his own life, he just happens to be around when I'm feeling down. Besides, I believe he and the icy Olivia are an item."

"Indeed."

Daniel's look was probing.

"I had hoped you would turn to me for support, I'm not a demonstrative man, just let me say, I'd like to be more than a friend, forgive me if that's presumptuous."

'More than a friend'.

She was stunned, she had never thought of Daniel romantically, although he could be considered very eligible.

Daniel…she shook her head, he was confident, bordering on arrogance, she felt no attraction towards him.

She pictured Quinlan's face, serious as he listened to her, his eyes alight with compassion. She shook her head, dispelling the image.

Deep in thought, she made her way to the Q.E.H, feeling at home as soon as she entered the lobby.

In nursing admin, she completed the necessary paperwork, then sought the linen room to be measured for uniform and have her photo taken for the name tag.

Back in admin she was seen by the assistant Director of Nursing, and with her choice of part time duty in the psychiatric unit, agreed to be available for orientation the next day.

She loved hospitals, the sense of purpose, the busy hum of activity, even the familiar smell, a compound of chemicals, and antiseptics.

Seeing a group of nurses walking towards the cafeteria, she joined them, taking her coffee to one of the many staff tables, now occupied by a red-headed girl in uniform.

"Civilian or staff member?" The registered nurse enquired pleasantly.

Gabrielle held out her hand. "Gabrielle Graham, I start tomorrow with orientation, then I'm in the psych unit."

"Josephine Gibson, Jo to my friends, I'm in Kids ward, hopefully temporarily, sick kids upset me."

"Same here, I haven't nursed children since I finished training ten years ago."

Jo, distracted, picked up her empty cup, her face suddenly flushed.

"May I?"

Connor's deep voice was obviously the cause of Jo's blushing confusion.

Gabrielle smiled, gesturing to the unoccupied chair. Jo with a brief glance at Quinlan stood.

"I'm due back, welcome to the Q.E.H." and smiling at Gabrielle, left.

Gabrielle was unable to resist a broad grin at Quinlan.

"The lady's smitten," amused at his 'no comment.'

Gradually, the cafeteria filled, an obvious meeting place for staff, and patient family members.

She finished her coffee. "I start tomorrow so I'll no doubt see you around."

"Oh, you can't stay for a few moments?"

She was aware that she and Quinlan were the object of some scrutiny.

"No, I must see Daniel before he leaves this afternoon."

"Leaves?"

" Yes, he's off to the States, Richard has been traced to New York."

"I see, may I phone you this evening?"

"Do."

Despite her outwardly cool manner, she experienced a surge of delight at the thought that she might see him tonight..

Her pulse raced when she looked at him. She acknowledged silently that her feelings for Richard had been lukewarm, compared with the rush of emotion she felt when with Connor. She wondered if he was aware of her attraction towards him..

Orientation occupied the following day; with several other new staff members she was given a tour of the three hundred-bedded hospital.

" I'll show you the ward you're rostered to, then Cas, Outpatients physio, and X ray, I don't want to confuse you, you'll find your way around in time," the R/n smiled.

Finally, theatres, and the surgical suites, which occupied the third floor. She wondered if Jo Gibson was on duty. She resolved to lunch in the cafeteria, and perhaps catch up with Jo.

The group returned to the classroom, for compulsory first aid and a video on health and safety practices. Later, orientation complete, she collected her uniform and identification tag, and took the lift to the second floor, intent on meeting the sister in charge of the psychiatric ward and looking at the duty roster.

She looked forward to meeting the ward staff, expecting to be welcomed. Initially, she had chosen to work part time, aware that the busy hospital was short-staffed, and would welcome a competent R/n.

In the ward, Sister Jenman waved her into the office.

"Sister Graham, so good to see you, I expect you want to look at the roster?"

Seated at the desk, Gabrielle wrote down her fortnight's roster, noting she was rostered for Monday, Wednesday, and Friday, preferring to work a late shift, at this stage, and on call if necessary.

More than she expected but prepared to accept it in the short term. Minutes later, walking back to the lift, she heard a female voice raised in protest.

'I don't care about that, make time.'

Chapter Seven

She was uncomfortably aware she had overheard the voices in Quinlan's office.

Olivia Sanders, eyes glittering, swept past, not acknowledging Gabrielle's nod of recognition, the door to Quinlan's office slamming in her wake.

She chose to use the stairs, unwilling to witness Quinlan's response to what would appear a lover's quarrel, should he follow Olivia. Eating supper that evening, she pondered Olivia's anger, feeling disquiet at the thought of Quinlan and Olivia Sanders intimately associated.

She smiled ruefully, he was an attractive acquaintance, no more. Perhaps they would become friends, although on reflection, she knew Olivia Sanders would not accept that notion with equanimity.

She had agreed to work a three on, four off roster, which included three late shifts, so she would cover Sister Jenman's time away from the ward. Monday, Wednesday, and Friday, 3.30pm to 11pm.

All things being equal, she would eventually be offered a full-time position. Until she started work, she determined to spend time looking for some clue to Richard's last few days in the house. Mid-morning, absorbed in her task and surrounded by the neat stacks of paperwork she had systematically looked through, she was startled by the doorbell.

She had forgotten Daniel's call the previous evening, and his request to see her before he left for the States.

Daniel was immaculate, his aftershave pleasant as he leaned to kiss her cheek.

"Not interrupting I hope?"

His broad frame filled the doorway.

"Sorting through Richard's paperwork, nothing of note so far."

Daniel followed her into the kitchen, watching as she filled the jug.

"Coffee? I haven't stopped since breakfast at seven, I could use a break."

"Gabrielle, I doubt you'll find anything, so far, the only mistake Richard has made is using his visa card and the traveler's cheques".

Hearing the tension in his voice, she paused, looking at him.

"Gabrielle, Richard's married."

Stunned, she watched as he pulled a chair from the table gently guiding her to sit.

"That's impossible, I would have known."

She took the linen handkerchief he proffered, wiping the tears that welled, repeating.

"Impossible…"

"Sadly, it's true, I spoke to his wife this morning."

Stricken, she stared.

"His wife that's… that's "

Daniel, familiar with the house, left the kitchen, returning several minutes later with a cut glass tumbler, his face troubled as he poured the contents into her coffee cup.

Wincing, she drank, feeling the alcohol burn her throat; she imagined Daniel's abrupt manner was fueled by anger.

"Married… he wasn't content with larceny, he planned on bigamy as well."

Daniel grimaced.

"So it would seem."

She laughed, the sound unnerving in the peaceful tranquility of the sunny kitchen.

"Crazy, none of it makes sense."

"Her name is Alexandra, she's a New Yorker, she met Richard there three years ago when he was in New York on business".

She pushed the cup away. Alexandra... Alex.

"He said he had problems on that trip, he was preoccupied and irritable when he came back."

She paused, remembering how Richard, previously so attentive and romantic, had pleaded pressure of work to explain his ill temper and lack of concentration. In the year since they had met, they had spent less than three months together, he in one continent, she in another; with his promise that when she moved to Australia, they would spend their life together.

Daniel remained silent, seeing her struggle to hold back tears.

"Does she know he's a thief, a would be bigamist, and a liar?"

Daniel nodded. "She's pregnant with their first child, she's resolved to stand by him."

"Pregnant?

That's beyond belief... and that he was married when I met him."

Her heart thundered in her chest, shuddering, she realised how close she had been to 'marrying' a married man. She finished the whisky, lightheaded with shock, hunger, and alcohol.

"My stomach's growling."

Daniel opened the fridge.

"A sandwich, how does that sound?"

"Great, if you can be bothered, I'm embarrassed to admit I'm hungry."

His back to her, voice husky, he said.

"Sweetie, there isn't anything I wouldn't do.... "

She interrupted. "Thank you, you're very.... considerate."

Inadequate, but the best she could manage, she wanted no more declarations of undying love, regardless of who made them. Daniel faced her, food forgotten momentarily.

"I didn't ask how long they'd been married, although from what Alexandra said, she sees little of him. She knows his business is based in Australia, she works in New York, for the law firm Raglan Pearce have had an association with since Malcolm started way back in the seventies."

"Her father is C.E.O of the firm, a mover and shaker. Richard has been our representative for six years or more; plenty of time to form relationships in that time."

Gabrielle grimaced. "What a prize fool I've been, believing everything he said, leaving my family and home to follow an illusion."

"Don't blame yourself, we've all been misled, he's a master manipulator, I've 'known' him for years and I still don't know him."

He handed a plate to her. "I must go, I 'll phone as soon as I can, in the meantime I think you're fortunate that he didn't stay to 'marry' you."

Quinlan's sentiments repeated. She walked him to the car.

"Stay in touch.

Back in the house, she rinsed the cups, hungry but disinterested in the sandwich Daniel had prepared.

Richard, married. She experienced the idea with no sense of loss; confused by her feelings.

She realised she had not known him, accepting the sophisticated, good-looking façade he presented, and willing to suspend her usual common sense self, seduced by his

 his smooth talk, his ability to create a persona based on his physical appeal and apparent wealth.

All lies and fraud, and she had considered herself blessed to be 'chosen' by him as his life partner; had wanted to believe he was her soul mate.

 Strangely, instead of despair, she felt relief, shocked by the understanding that she was free of him. Why had she not realised how shallow he was?

 Perhaps, since meeting Connor, the comparison between the two men was impossible to ignore.

Thinking herself her own woman, she had been a gullible partner in Richard's devious, clever manipulation. For the brief months of their relationship, he had changed her image of the person she believed herself to be.

How trustingly she had offered herself to this stranger, had allowed him to define who she was. She had not realised what he wanted was not who she was. She had willingly abetted his definition of her, whilst presenting himself as honest, trustworthy, and caring. Wanting to believe, she ignored her instincts.

'More fool me', she thought wryly.

On reflection, she realised she was not in love with Richard, intrigued, attracted, bemused, yes, love, no.

Love was the bond between her parents, respect, trust, friendship, the quiet confidence of a mature proven partnership. Each secure enough to have their own identity, and choosing to be together because they valued qualities in each other, enriched by the years together.

She was angry that she had not questioned the speed with which the romance occurred. Her parent's concern was unheeded, she was a levelheaded adult, she knew how to conduct her life.

A flawed sense of security had allowed this shallow, devious man to turn her life upside down.

Given the knowledge of Richard's deceit she would not stay in the house.

He had become a stranger. Knowing he was married, that he would soon be a father, was shocking.

She wanted no part of him, shuddering to think how willingly she had stepped into the deception that was his life.

It took a short time to pack her suitcases and check nothing was left behind. The Jaguar would allow mobility until she bought a car. Perhaps May could spare some time to show her the local car yards.

May answered the phone immediately, asking if she had news of Richard, and agreeing to accompany her that afternoon.

With a sense of relief, she locked the front door and stowed the suitcases in the car, she would keep the house keys until she returned the Jaguar.

May was waiting, the front door opening before Gabriel exited the Jaguar. May lead her into the lounge, where there were several baskets, full of balls of wool. Every imaginable pastel colour. Blues, pinks, mauves, green., Gabrielle thought they were entrancing.

"I'm interrupting your work."

May beamed at Gabrielle.

"I'm crocheting a shawl for my daughter. Do you knit or crochet?"

Gabrielle shook her head.

" I'd love to learn."

"Perhaps I can teach you?"

Gabrielle smiled. "Thank you, I'd appreciate that."

May said. "I wondered how you were, and if Mr. Pearce had been in touch?"

"May, he's in America, he won't be back, I'm afraid your instinct was correct."

" He's done something very... well... disastrous really, I won't stay in the house, and I need my own car, I'd be glad if you'll show me where the car yards are?"

"I'm so sorry to hear that."

May's kind face was troubled.

"Will you have a cup of tea or coffee, before we go?"

"Thank you, no, I'm beginning to speed with all the caffeine I've drunk in the last couple of days."

She laughed, and was heartened to see May grin in response,

"No good crying over spilt milk, my mother would say."

"I'm ready to go if you are, Miss Graham."

"Gabrielle, please, you aren't in Richard's employ now, I'm glad to have you as a friend."

May drove them to the main road where several car dealers were located. Gabrielle was very specific about the car she wanted, and neither salesman in the first two yards had the Toyota she sought.

In the third yard, there were three Toyotas all older and in poorer condition than she was willing to accept.

May took her arm as they left the yard. "Morgan's on North Road, might have what you want, turn left at the next set of lights, they're on the left."

Morgan's had a huge selection of cars, and   the young salesman took the two women around the yard, pointing to a group of vehicles, all freshly detailed.

"There are a couple of Toyotas here that might suit you, the later model has just been traded, only three thousand on the odometer, in great condition and with a year's warranty."

Eagerly the salesman showed the car's immaculate interior. "How about a test drive?"

The car purred into life without fault. "Smooth as silk," enthused the salesman, and Gabrielle agreed, after a short trip along the main road.

She was pleased with her choice, and back at the yard the salesman accepted her personal cheque, having photocopied her driving licence, and passport. Since May knew the area well, it was agreed that Gabrielle would follow her back to the house in the Toyota. She was thankful, two of her goals accomplished, she had a job, and reliable transport, her next priority was accommodation.

 Again, May was resourceful, she had a guest room Gabrielle could use whilst looking for a flat or apartment. She agreed on condition that May accepted financial reimbursement, a satisfactory outcome for both women. She was mindful of Richard's shortcomings; she would not take advantage of May's generous nature.

The guest room was small but adequate in the short term. May had a tray with tea and biscuits prepared when Gabrielle returned to the sitting room.

"The room is small, but you're welcome to stay until you decide on a plan of action, I must say, I'll enjoy your company."

She knew May's only son was married and lived in Perth, and that she only saw her grandchildren at Christmas. She had confided that her son wanted her to move to Perth.

"I was born in Robe in the southeast. I've lived in South Australia all my life; I married and had my son in this house. All my friends are here, I'm too old to pick up and move, much as I love my son and the family."

Mr. Burns had left May after their child was born, she confided.

"We were too young for the responsibility of marriage, and a child. He said I spent too much time caring for the baby, he spent all his time in the pub, so I learned how to look after my son. Now I realise, what I hoped for in a partner when I was twenty, wasn't what I wanted at thirty, and now I'm fifty, I've become too independent, or so my friends tell me."

Smiling at her, May said. "Which isn't to say I wouldn't welcome a gentle, caring man in my life, it's just not the be all and end all now."

Gabrielle accepted a mug of tea, her face thoughtful.

 "I think women are 'programmed' by society, to believe marriage is a must, a validation of 'self'."

"The 'other half,' I don't see myself as a 'half', waiting for someone to make me 'whole'. "

"Even so, I allowed a stranger to deceive me, not seeing beyond the good looks, and glamorous lifestyle. May. I'm starting to believe the 'if it looks too good to be true,' maxim, and, on a practical note, I need a visa since there won't be a marriage."

"Mr. Pearce seemed the perfect gentleman, whatever difficulty he had only happened in the last few weeks. Trust, Gabrielle, if we distrusted people we know, life would be a grim business."

" Ring immigration, you have a job and no dependents, so you shouldn't have a problem with getting a work visa"

Chapter Eight

The day passed uneventfully. After the phone call to immigration, she was assured she could apply for a work visa, and that the forms would be sent to her. It was good news; she could start looking for an apartment. She liked May, but needed her own space.

The following day, Thursday, the two made a list of real estate agents, rental properties were plentiful, and she had no difficulty finding a neat two-bedroom house within walking distance of the hospital.

The tenant had three days left on the lease.

"Moving to Melbourne."

Explained the real estate agent, knocking on the front door, and taking a key from his pocket.

"He knows I'm showing the house, he said he'll tidy up."

The house was larger than it appeared from the outside, they were shown through the hall to the kitchen where French doors led to a small courtyard garden.

Perched on the dividing wall, a ginger cat eyed them disdainfully, then continued grooming.

"Even a cat."

The real estate agent grinned.

Of all the houses Gabrielle and May had inspected that day, this was by far the most appealing and they returned to the office to make the necessary transactions. In three days, the agent promised she could move in.

That evening, she took May to dinner. "A small way of saying 'thank you' for being so supportive".

May beamed. "Hopefully, a new beginning so you can leave the past behind."

Gabrielle had kept the key to Richard's house. Leaving the restaurant she wondered if any messages had been left on the answering machine.

The house was still and dark, May shivered, reaching for the hall light switch.

"What's to become of the house, will it be sold?"

"Richard won't be back, so it depends on what Daniel decides I suppose."

Entering the library, she rewound the tape and pressed 'play.'

Daniel's voice, surprisingly loud in silence, greeted her. He had seen Richard and Alexandra, and been assured that the money would be repaid. Richard had written and she could expect his letter in a day or two.

 Richard regretted what had occurred, the letter would explain his actions.

'I'll be back day after tomorrow sweetie, keep your chin up.'

Daniel paused, then, his voice soft.

 'I'm looking forward to seeing you.'

She erased the message and joined May in the sitting room.

 "Daniel left a message, Richard won't be back, no surprise there, it would seem all will be resolved."

May smiled. "That's good news, isn't it?"

"For the law firm, yes. I'm ambivalent, I can hear my parents saying 'darling, come home'.

"I'm resolved to stay for a year at least, I have a job, somewhere to live, and the opportunity to work and explore Australia."

"Good for you, and, Gabrielle, any way I can help out you only have to ask."

The weekend sped by, spent getting the flat orderly, and on Monday morning she arrived at the Q.E.H, eagerly anticipating her first day on the psychiatric ward.

Sister Jenman was in the office, preparing for the handover.

Smiling, she pulled a chair forward.

"Welcome, once we've had the report, I'll take you round the ward. No one for 'shock' this morning, Wednesday's our E.C.T. (electro convulsive therapy) day".

Both night nurses and day staff waited for the handover.

The ward housed eighteen patients, it was an open ward, treating patients with illnesses that did not require nursing in a locked ward.

She spent the day introducing herself to the patients and reading notes.

Sister Jenman had allotted several patients to her care, as well as the responsibility of overseeing the student nurses on the ward and giving medications.

Looking at the admission book, she saw diagnoses of depression, obsessive compulsive, and anxiety disorder, personality disorders, Bipolar disorder, and anorexia. Each patient saw the psychiatrist on a weekly basis, and currently, only one elderly woman was being treated with electroconvulsive therapy for her depressive illness.

The first day on duty passed quickly. She introduced herself again to the group, then gave a brief account of herself, inviting each patient to share appropriate insights about their life, and the circumstances which brought them to the psychiatric unit.

Her suggestion of an informal 'self-help' group discussion hour was approved by Sister Jenman, and after lunch, Gabrielle, with eight interested patients, entered the therapy room

Sitting quietly in the group, she was able to develop an understanding of each person, who was shy, who more assertive.

Two patients did not speak, both teenagers, suffering anorexia. She knew from previous experience that not all patients were able to share personal details initially.

Trust was an issue. She spoke of boundaries, and outlined what positive benefits a group of supportive individuals offered if successfully managed.

She emphasised the importance of honesty, and respect for each other's feelings, whether or not the group agreed about the subject matter.

The last fifteen minutes were spent teaching relaxation techniques, so vital in helping with the stresses of day-to-day life.

At the end of the hour, she thanked the group, there would be a notice on the 'info' board about the next group meeting; any patient who felt they would benefit from one-on-one counselling was encouraged to ask her.

That afternoon, she left the hospital gratified that her first shift had been productive.

Walking to the car park, she noticed Olivia Sanders deep in conversation with Quinlan. Swiftly, she unlocked the Toyota, and threw her bag into the rear seat. She preferred not to confront them together.

"Gabrielle, not so fast."

Olivia stood glowering, as Quinlan moved towards the Toyota. Embarrassed, Gabrielle glanced in the mirror knowing her face was flushed. She wound the window down smiling at him.

"Connor, how are you?"

In his long white coat, he was undeniably gorgeous.

"I'm well, how was your first day?"

Casually, he leaned into the car, in the distance, she saw Olivia turn to look at them before she disappeared into the hospital.

"Good, the staff are excellent, I have a group of patients, nothing I can't manage."

"Several of them are my patients, you'll see me in the ward from time to time."

She nodded; patient care was something they could talk about without her heart thumping erratically.

"Finished for the day?"

She nodded again.

"On my way home, I moved into a house in Lisburne Avenue."

"That calls for a celebratory drink, or better still, dinner?" He raised his eyebrows enquiringly.

"Sounds good, I'm still unpacking boxes, so yes, dinner is definitely a goer."

"You're learning the lingo."

She laughed. "Why not? "

"How's seven this evening, I see my last patient at four, and I have a few notes to dictate?"

Smiling, he straightened and turned back to the hospital.

She drove to the flat, thinking about Olivia and the relationship she so obviously had with Quinlan, and wondering at Quinlan's reason for asking her to dinner.

Surely he was being compassionate, offering the hand of friendship knowing how traumatic her first weeks in Australia had been.

She felt a twinge of regret at the thought of Quinlan interested in friendship only. Richard's absence caused her no pain. Anger and perhaps embarrassment at her willing acceptance of him, and an awareness that she didn't miss him, and was glad he was no longer part of her life.

Quinlan however,….she parked the Toyota in the drive, musing as she entered the house, Quinlan was a man she respected, honest, compassionate, and, she smiled, shaking her head at her wayward thoughts, he was powerfully attractive.

She recalled the heart stopping feeling of being held close, breathing in the heady pipe tobacco, cologne, and undeniably masculine scent of him.

Enough daydreaming, she had time to unpack the remaining boxes before Quinlan arrived, vowing she would not intrude on Olivia's relationship with Quinlan.

He had kissed her. True, perhaps the whisky played some part in that, even so it would be a long time before she allowed any man into her life regardless of his appeal.

That evening she enjoyed Quinlan's company, aware that other women in the restaurant gazed at him with interest.

His engaging smile and complete attention to her was undeniably charming, the thought of Richard and the last few miserable weeks forgotten.

After dinner he suggested they leave his car at the restaurant, and walk in the Botanic Gardens beside the River Torrens. As they moved closer to the gardens they heard music playing and saw lights twinkling on the riverbank.

Quinlan placed his hand on her shoulder guiding her down the bank.

"The local choir give concerts here, Dr Bryant sings with them 'though I've never heard him sing."

She was surprised to see a large crowd, some sitting on the grass, others on folding chairs. Quinlan stopped, taking his jacket off.

"The grass is fairly dry; we can sit here if you like?"

She sat beside him, listening to the familiar carols. Each of the thirty or so singers held a lantern, more for effect than to read the music.

"That's Mike, second on the left at the back, he has a nice tenor."

She watched Mike Bryan, agreeing he had a pleasant tenor voice.

The choirmaster turned to the crowd.

"The last carol, folks, 'Holy Night', please join in."

Quinlan stood, holding her hand to help her up.

She listened to Quinlan's surprisingly good baritone; Mike Bryant wasn't the only talented doctor on the Q. E. H's staff. Quinlan grinned down at her, still holding her hand.

"I sang with the choir for several years, before Clare died, Mike joined the month I left; it was good fun, and they always welcome new members."

"Connor, enjoying the evening?"

Olivia Sanders, lovely in casual slacks and Aran sweater, smiled at Quinlan, nodding an acknowledgement of Gabrielle.

Mike Bryant put his arm around Olivia's shoulder.

"Quinlan, enjoy the concert?"

"We arrived at the end, Mike, this is Gabrielle Graham, she started work in the psych unit this week."

Bryant smiled at Gabrielle, "That's good news, I'll no doubt see you in the hospital."

Olivia smiled again at Quinlan, then gave Gabrielle a look with no warmth in it.

"See you tomorrow, Connor, don't forget our lunch date."

Seated again in Quinlan's car, she broke the silence, thanking him for a pleasant evening. Silently, they drove to the house, and she waited while he exited the car to open the door for her.

"Gabrielle, Olivia's... we... "

"Connor, no explanations are necessary, it's none of my business."

"I want to tell you.... "

She opened the door. "Thank you again, I'll see you tomorrow."

After several minutes, she heard Quinlan drive away. She prepared for bed, regretting that she had responded to him by ignoring him.

Since she had no intention of getting involved with him, why did she feel a keen sense of disappointment at the thought of Olivia's relationship with him?

Her last thought before sleep claimed her was that she would avoid Quinlan and Olivia Sanders whenever possible.

On duty that afternoon she noted there had been an admission the previous afternoon.

Sister Jenman requested that Gabrielle included a mid-twenties man in her patient group. His medical notes were en route from the psychiatric facility he had been treated at previously.

The afternoon passed quickly, she was kept busy giving medications, holding her group therapy session, and writing notes.

Chapter Nine

She had packed her lunch, preferring not to eat in the canteen, and at twelve thirty p.m, made her way to a secluded area in the hospital gardens.

 In the branches of a nearby silver birch, several parrots pecked at catkins, as she watched fascinated.

The bird life here was amazing, in England, she had seen flocks of pigeons, sparrows, gulls, but nothing as spectacular as the brightly coloured parrots, and varieties of honeyeaters she enjoyed watching now.

Absorbed, she was startled by Olivia Sanders' voice.

"Miss Graham, I was hoping to see you."

Gabrielle made room for Olivia, turning to face her, smiling.

"Please call me Gabrielle."

"Doctor Quinlan is off limits, Miss Graham, I trust I make myself clear."

For a full minute, Gabrielle stared at the lovely face, made less appealing by the cold smile.

"That's not for you to say, surely?"

"Oh, but it is, he has no need of you in his life."

Gabrielle retreated, stunned by the venomous glare. She wondered if Quinlan knew Olivia was capable of such hostility.

As swiftly as she had appeared, Olivia was gone. Gabrielle remained seated, appalled by the brief exchange.

She was thankful when 11pm came, her next day on duty was Friday; she needed time away from the hospital to make sense of the incident with Olivia. She drove to May's house, glad when May welcomed her with a smile.

Gabrielle sat at the kitchen table, while May filled the jug, and laid a tray, taking a sponge from the cupboard.

"This is freshly baked; will you try a piece?"

"Thanks, May."

"Gabrielle, tell me to mind my own business, you do seem rather down 'though."

"Nothing I can't deal with, something at work that shook me."

May sat opposite her, placing the mug of tea on the table .

"Anything you want to share?"

"I've been told very bluntly, not to become friendly with a psychologist who works at the hospital."

"Nothing wrong with being friendly, and the psychologist is male?"

Gabrielle laughed. "Very, that's why I've been told to stay away."

May nodded. "This is the surgeon you mentioned, Olivia?"

"Yes, she's an orthopaedic surgeon, who looks like a supermodel, Daniel completely lost the plot when he saw her, she's stunning."

" Will you comply?"

Despite herself, Gabrielle laughed again.

"I'll stay out of their way, I've no intention of making life even more difficult for myself. It seems odd, 'though, to be so hostile, when Connor and I have nothing more than a casual friendship."

"Perhaps not so casual, if you've been told to keep away."

That night in the quiet comfort of the flat, she recalled the malice in Olivia's eyes, wondering again at the relationship between Quinlan and Olivia.

Early on Friday morning, Daniel phoned, intent on seeing her that day. She tidied the flat, preparing lunch for him, apprehensive without knowing why.

Daniel arrived promptly at midday, handing her a cellophane wrapped bouquet of exquisite roses and kissing her cheek.

Seated on the sofa, he gazed at her.

"It's good to see you, and such a relief to be home. I brought Richard's letter with me if you want to read it now?"

"Later, you saw him, then?"

"Oh yes, met his wife, and her father, Richard told them he had 'borrowed' from the firm, his father-in-law agreed to give Richard a job, the money will be recovered, all in all, he's a lucky man."

"His wife supports the decision?"

"She's not at all what I expected."

" I think her pregnancy and the fact that she and her family are Catholics, means she won't divorce him, she accepts that he's been deceitful; she made it plain he can't afford to put a foot wrong; an admirable young woman."

They ate lunch, Gabrielle listening to Daniel's account of the whirlwind trip and Richard's seemingly genuine repentance.

"Gabrielle, I know this has been tough on you, I'm thankful that it's been resolved and that the firm will continue as before with Dad managing the trust accounts."

"I'm glad, too, although how Richard will pay back what he stole is beyond me."

"His father-in-law will send a bank cheque, and Richard will spend the next six or seven years working to pay the debt."

"Richard's fortunate his wife's family are decent, law-abiding folk."

She took the dishes to the sink and busied herself with the percolator. "Coffee?"

"Please, how's the new job, is it what you expected?"

An hour passed, before Daniel rose.

 "I must go, will you have dinner with me this evening, there's still a lot to tell you."

She agreed, choosing to meet him at the restaurant near the hospital.

 She was fast learning that having her own transport gave her independence, she could come and go as she pleased. She smiled, albeit grimly, at the thought; Richard had taught her an invaluable lesson, reliance on herself, and her instincts.

On Friday, she worked a 3.30 to 11.30pm shift. Several of the patients had left the ward for the weekend, four of her group remained, among them, the young man admitted on her last day on.

 He was a nice-looking man, tall with an engaging smile. His notes were in the trolley, and she read his discharge letter from the unit he had spent several months at. She noted his diagnosis, personality disorder.

His notes were voluminous; an abusive home environment, in foster care at thirteen, then a juvenile detention centre, for setting fire to the home of his foster parents.

With another boy, Adam had absconded from the unit, living on the streets until he was caught shoplifting, and returned to detention. Medication and psychological counselling had failed to halt his impulsive, self-destructive behaviour.

She wondered at the diagnosis of severe antisocial personality disorder, she had nursed other patients with a similar diagnosis; knowing how easy it was to be charmed into forgetting how untrustworthy and destructive such people were; not guided by moral principles, cold and scheming.

They easily mimicked normal human emotions, not, in any way feeling the emotion. They were capable of committing horrendous crimes, with complete detachment and a lack of remorse.

She noted that Adam was in care of the Guardianship Board, deemed in need of his affairs and finances being managed by the Board.

He requested access to his wallet, which was locked along with other personal items in the ward safe.

"What are your plans, Adam?"

Smiling beguilingly, he leaned across the desk, his face inches from hers.

"I just need my wallet, and I'll be out of your way."

"How do you plan on spending the afternoon?"

"Nosy, aren't we?"

"Adam, you know well enough you have a limit on the amount of money you're allowed on any given day, what are you doing later?"

"If it's all the same to you I'm going into town, I need some stuff, and a counter meal would be a change from the crap we get here."

She had unlocked the safe and taken a large hospital envelope with Adam's name on it.

"Twenty dollars, Adam, you must tell Sister Jenman if you need a staff member to accompany you on a shopping trip."

"It's my bloody money, twenty dollars won't get me far."

"Far enough, do you want it?"

'Sister, be a sport, can't we keep quiet about this? I need a hundred or it's not worth going out."

"Then, Adam, you must stay here."

"Oh f…. "He snatched the twenty dollar note, scowling.

"Do you want your bus pass?"

"F… you and the bus pass."

'Charming,' Gabrielle thought as the man stalked out into the corridor.

Adam Morrison was not the first patient to become verbally abusive, when thwarted, and he would not be the last.

Sociopaths…she was very familiar with the manipulative, cold, self-centered characteristics, the complete disregard for others, and the lack of empathy and of conscience.

This outrageous behaviour was accepted by the patient as permissible.

She knew from long experience that people with sociopathic tendencies could be very charming and utterly skillful in persuading others to trust them.

Reflecting, she thought that in many ways the person with sociopathic traits was very much like an indulged small child, wanting instant gratification of whichever whim occurred.

Unlike a small child who perhaps became 'socialised,' the behaviour continued and too often the sociopathic adult was a familiar part of the psychiatric community.

She remembered that, as a postgraduate student nurse, she was asked to accompany a group of five patients on an outing into the town of Norwich in England. The day was mild, spring weather, and the group set forth with much anticipation.

The bus took them to the town centre, where they wandered around the shops and stopped for coffee in a small café in the mall.

Three of the patients were female, all with a diagnosis of schizophrenia, which was managed relatively adequately with medication.

Of the remaining two male patients, one suffered from obsessive compulsive disorder, and the other, Raymond, a teenager of some eighteen or nineteen years, had a diagnosis of sociopathic personality disorder. The morning passed swiftly enjoyed by all.

Chapter Ten

At lunchtime Raymond suggested eating their packed lunch in the Botanic gardens, all in favour of the idea.

Lunch finished; the group were entertained by feeding the ducks with crusts from the sandwiches.

After twenty minutes of this activity, she realised Raymond had left the group and the remaining four had no idea where he was. she hurried them back along the path they had taken earlier, with no success in sighting Raymond.

This was disastrous, she had no idea where to look or how to proceed, given she had the welfare of four other patients to consider.

She could not leave them sitting on a park bench trusting they would not wander away. Fortunately the dilemma was resolved. Several people walked towards the group, speaking loudly.

She heard someone say. "We should tell the park attendant, that's disgusting behaviour."

"Pardon me, you haven't seen a young man---.

"If he's with you, dear, you need to take him home before he gets himself into more trouble."

She led the group in the direction of pointing fingers.

Hastening past the shrubs bordering the shallow lake, she was appalled to see Raymond, soaking, in the middle of the lake, bending to pick up coins thrown in the water, a plaque dedicated the 'wishing well' to park users.

Raymond ignored her, intent on filling his pockets with ill-gotten money.

He did, however, raise his head at the shout of the park attendant who demanded to know.

'What the bloody hell did he think he was doing?'

To say she was embarrassed was to master understatement.

She introduced herself, telling the attendant that the group were patients in her care, she 'deeply regretted the incident, Raymond had wandered off.... '

"Take the buggers back where they came from."

(Raymond was grinning, totally unfazed by being marched out of the lake by the park attendant manager).

Gabrielle was humiliated, a crowd had gathered, attracted by the noise, and Raymond took great pleasure in the attention, grinning and bowing.

Several among the crowd applauded, inciting him to further display.

A skilled acrobat, he easily slipped from the park attendant's grasp, and performed several impressive cartwheels, scattering coins as he spun.

She frowned at the memory. Relaying the incident to the other students later, she learned she had been 'set up', the ward staff knew of Raymond's unpredictable behaviour and enjoyed students panic at the inevitable chaos an outing with Raymond brought.

She thought the ward staff's behaviour was outrageous, Raymond had a diagnosed psychiatric disorder.

What was the staff's excuse for putting an unsuspecting student and a group of vulnerable patients at risk?

Gabrielle thought it strange that professional adults would behave in such a manner.

At 8.30pm it was apparent Raymond had absconded; she rang nursing admin to report his absence.

The police would be informed, and fate would take its course. In an open ward, patients could and did take advantage of the fact that staff were busy and unable to monitor them constantly.

Most abided by hospital policy; Raymond was not among that number.

His notes indicated he had left other psych hospital grounds without permission on numerous occasions, escorted back by several policemen.

She had no doubt the same would happen.

Taking responsibility for someone bent on misbehaving was no easy task, particularly when that person was in the care of the Guardianship Board.

At 11.30pm, she handed over to night staff, ensuring Raymond was listed as absent without leave. preparing for bed, she was thankful that her first week of work had been relatively uneventful.

Deeply asleep, she was startled into consciousness by the shrill ringing of the phone beside the bed.

"Hello?"

The sound of breathing alerted her.

"Hello, this is..."

No, better not give her name or phone number. She replaced the receiver, the travel clock showed 2.30am, whoever had phoned must have the wrong number.

She heard again the sound of someone breathing, if it was a misdial surely the caller would apologise?

Again, the phone rang, and she listened to the harsh sound of breathing.

Without speaking, she pulled the connection from the wall, now let whomever it was harass her.

Fully awake, she reached for her robe, and walked downstairs, checking that the curtains were drawn in each room, and the house securely locked.,

She was puzzled rather than alarmed by the incident. Perhaps the person or persons who had leased the flat before her, had angered someone sufficiently enough to cause problems.

She was a newcomer, not well known; little reason to suppose the silent phone call was directed at her.

Heartened by the thought, she returned to bed, lying awake for some time before falling into an uneasy sleep.

She was awakened by the ring of the doorbell, putting on her robe she hastened downstairs blinking in the sunlight.

Daniel, immaculate in slacks and open necked shirt stood looking at her, obviously surprised at her deshabille.

"Late night?"

He followed her into the kitchen, sitting at the table and watching her fill the jug.

"You could say that; a phone call at some ungodly hour this morning."

"Not trouble, I hope?"

"Some clown thinking it amusing to breathe heavily into the phone."

"What?"

"That reminds me, the phone is disconnected, I won't be a moment."

Downstairs, Daniel had taken mugs from the cupboard.

"Gabrielle, perhaps a silent number would be advisable, I don't like the idea of you alone here without the phone available."

"I don't think the call was directed at me; I don't know anyone who has reason to dislike me."

"Even so, promise you'll think about it?"

"What brings you here so early, Daniel?"

Looking at her watch, she was surprised to see it was 12.45pm.

"Good grief, I had no idea it was so late, I promised May I'd shop with her at the Central market.

Daniel frowned. "I hoped you'd spend the day with me, I have a lot to tell you."

"I'm pretty well flat out this weekend unless your news is vitally important?"

He shook his head. "No, just general news about my trip, and I wondered what you thought of Richard's letter?"

Richard's letter, still upstairs in her jacket pocket.

"I forgot about it, I worked a 'late' and the phone call woke me. Daniel, you must excuse me, I want to shower and get dressed."

Daniel grimaced, "Gabrielle, must I make an appointment to see you?"

Embarrassed, she gulped a mouthful of hot tea.

" Daniel, I can offer friendship, am I being presumptuous in thinking you want more than that?"

To her surprise, he blushed, standing up so quickly, his tea spilled onto the table.

"I'll let you get ready, will you phone if you need me? "

"I'm a big girl, Daniel, I really can take care of myself."

Showering, she realised he had not replied to her question, she liked Daniel, friendship, certainly…. lover, definitely not. Recalling the letter, she retrieved it from her pocket. Shaking her head, she studied Richard's familiar writing.

'Dear Gabrielle, by now you know all there is to know about the embezzlement, and the fact that I'm married to Alexandra and we're expecting a baby in six weeks.

I could say I'm sorry, however, that wouldn't begin to describe the pain I feel, about cheating on Alexandra, and on you. Please know that the worry about the money I stole was so overwhelming, nothing else mattered, even the damage I did to you.

I hope you can learn to forgive me. You are a remarkable woman, and I loved you, in my own selfish way. Take care of yourself, my wish for you, is that one day soon, you will meet a man who is worthy of you. Love, Richard.'

In thirty minutes she was in the car on her way to May's house.

The Central Market was huge and undercover. Stalls side by side, sold every variety of fruit and vegetables in season. Cheese, bread, seafood, including shark, and octopus; and gourmet produce. Food courts, small stalls with preloved books and clothes, and in the air the heady aroma of barbequed sausages, and hamburgers.

"Apart from the fruit and vegetables, you can find homemade produce, and all the ingredients locally supplied from farms around here," said May.

Gabrielle bought three punnets of raspberries, and browsed through books, on the stall presided over by the woman she knew as Richard's neighbour.

"How are you? Richard back from wherever it was? "

Smiling, she used a recipe book to distract the woman.

"Not yet, I'll take this, thanks."

"Two dollars; first time at the market?"

"Yes, May's been here many times, I've just discovered it."

Walking away, she told May that the stall holder lived in the house next to Richard's. Looking at the book, she smiled at the title. 'Cooking with herbs.'

"Handy, I had no idea what it was, I didn't want to tell an outright lie and say he was home, or tell people he won't be back, so I mumble."

May laughed. "That'll work, you don't have to tell anyone your business."

Gabrielle gazed around the market. Many stalls displayed gifts for Christmas, knitted teddy bears, homemade chocolates, and baskets filled with a variety of potted plants, fruit, and biscuits.

She had forgotten Christmas was ten days away, thinking that if Richard was here, they would be anticipating their wedding day, and the honeymoon in Barbados. With a start, she realised May had spoken.

"May, I was daydreaming, did you mention lunch?"

May nodded. "I love the C.W.A. lunches, the ladies raise funds for the old peoples' home by making sandwiches and cakes, my shout."

The hall was filled, several tables were set up on the lawn outside the library, and May placed her purchases on a chair.

"Gabrielle, stay here, I'll get us something to eat."

As May walked away, Gabrielle thought how different she was from the person she had been prior to coming to Australia. May joined her, carrying a tray on which sandwiches and small cakes were arranged.

"After this, I must finish the rest of my shopping, the cherries are beautiful this year, it's a family tradition to have a basket of tropical fruit, but I can never resist the cherries."

" I never come here without buying wool either."

May unwrapped the sandwiches, offering them to her.

"What plans do you have, you're not on duty I hope?"

Gabrielle smiled. "May, I've spent more Christmases on duty than I care to think about; in fact given the circumstances, working seems like a brilliant idea."

"You're more than welcome to spend the day with us."

Gabrielle calculated aloud. "Christmas day is on Saturday, ten days from now, I'll volunteer to work a shift. I know several married R/ns who would prefer to be home with their family; so I could work either the early or the late shift."

"Then spend some time with us?"

"May, I'd like that. I'll see Sister Jenman and let you know if I'm working."

"Incidentally, what do you think of this?"

May read the letter, then gave it to Gabrielle. "You dodged a bullet."

"Not the first time that's been said."

By six p.m, most stall owners were packing up, ready to leave the market.

Both May and Gabrielle had made several trips to their cars with purchases, looking forward to a quick visit to Chinatown, and planning to spend more time there after Christmas. Gabrielle, ready to head home, hugged May.

"I'll let you know if I'm working, May, thanks for today, I love the market."

May grinned, and with a wave, drove away. Gabrielle stopped at the mall, she would take a gift basket for May's family, and for May, something more personal.

Within minutes she had bought an exquisite teapot, cup and saucer, Staffordshire ware, which were gift wrapped for her.

Chapter Eleven

The house was quiet after the bustle of the market, she kicked off her shoes, after unloading her purchases from the car.

She had bought a book for Daniel, 'Antiques through the Ages,' she knew he was interested in antiques, and it was an impersonal 'safe' gift.

He could not read anything into the present, as perhaps he might if she gave him male toiletries, a tie, or something that indicated she was familiar with his tastes.

Smiling, she glanced through the book, stopping at a page with photographs of four poster beds.

Richard was sharing his bed, not a four poster, perhaps, but a bed, nevertheless.

She frowned, surprised at the thought. She felt not the slightest twinge of regret or jealousy, if anything, merely a sense of relief, knowing that chapter of her life had ended.

Sister Jenman, not surprisingly, welcomed Gabrielle's offer to work on Christmas day.

"Do you prefer a late or an early?"

"An early, if that's all right?"

"That will give us two R/ns on in the morning, and Sister Delaney and I on the late; I had last Christmas off, so I'm on this year."

Smiling at Gabrielle, Jenman penciled the change on the roster.

"Thanks for that, I don't like asking the R/ns with families to work an extra shift."

"I enjoy working on Christmas day; perhaps this morning I can take a few patients out shopping?"

"Excuse me, Sister."

Both R/ns looked at the student hovering at the door, behind her, two police officers in their familiar uniform.

"Good afternoon, Sisters, thought you'd like to know we caught up with Adam Burge, he's in custody at the station."

Adam had been apprehended by police, as he exited a house with stolen cash, and several visa cards.

"We'll return him this afternoon, if you can arrange the transfer to Park Bay; I'll phone before we leave the station."

Park Bay was a 'secure' psychiatric hospital, with locked wards which held patients who had committed criminal offences, but were suffering psychiatric disorders and therefore not incarcerated.

Sister Jenman sighed. "I don't know how many times he's been caught stealing, what a waste of a young life."

"Not for want of folks trying to help him, Sister; he carried on as if Constable Wright was the culprit, no remorse at all."

"That's the nature of his illness, Sergeant."

"A swift kick in the rear would sort him out." Constable Wright responded, grinning at her.

"Park Bay might not have a bed, Sergeant, and he can't be transferred here, he'd go 'walkabout' again."

"Won't take up any more of your time, Sister, I'll phone later, won't hurt young Burge to spend some 'quiet time' in the cells."

After both men had gone, Jenman closed the door, and took Adam's notes from the trolley.

"He's a worry, thankfully he didn't assault anyone this time."

Gabrielle was aware that Burge had a previous history of 'occasioning bodily harm.'

At eighteen, he had punched an elderly woman, as she fought to keep her bag. The local newspaper's account of the woman's distress prompted a huge response from the community.

Most householders believed 'whipping was too good for him.'

Gabrielle knew physical punishment would cause Adam Burge to become more vengeful, and no doubt exacerbate his behaviour. People with sociopathic disorders showed no regard for the rights of others.

Adam displayed the typical irresponsible, aggressive attitude, the inability to learn from previous experience, the lack of regard for his personal safety, that she knew to be indicative of the sociopathic personality. The fact that Burge abused alcohol and 'weed', (marijuana), exacerbated his problems.

"Will I take my group out; we can be back late afternoon?"

"Why not, I'll get some cash for you, perhaps enough for coffee and some shopping, you have five in your group I think?"

Only three of Gabrielle's patients took the opportunity to leave the hospital, several from other groups asked to be taken shopping. She agreed if Sister Jenman had no objection.

Eventually, with a group of six, each carrying a purse or wallet for their cash, they boarded the bus into town.

She knew the group would attract attention from visitors, residents used to patients taking the bus from the hospital, accepted them, visitors more apprehensive.

The afternoon passed smoothly, and it was with a sense of quiet contentment that she entered the house when her shift was over.

The following day, Gabrielle had six patients for group therapy, all diagnosed with O.C.D. Obsessive Compulsive Disorder. Many suffering from this distressing disorder were intelligent, well-educated people.

She introduced herself to the mixed group, telling them, that she was English, here in Adelaide to learn how Australian hospitals functioned.

She spoke briefly about the disorder, saying it was recognized as an anxiety disorder, forcing the sufferer to have compulsive or obsessive thoughts and behaviours, performed in a ritualistic way to quell their anxiety.

Obsessions were intrusive and recurrent mental pictures or impulses, which were often sexually inappropriate, caused distress and anxiety.

She explained that compulsions were the actions that the sufferer felt compelled to carry out.

Repetitive cleansing rituals, counting, hoarding, constant checking, an example being, that the stove had, indeed, been turned off, the door had been locked.

Religious obsessions, concerning blasphemy, or morality.

She knew that each individual knew exactly what she meant, their lives chaotic, because they spent each and every day, often well into the night, performing rituals.

Gabrielle emphasized the fact that sufferers of O.C.D hated the affliction, unlike those who overate, gambled, or engaged in numerous sexual affairs, deriving pleasure from such activities.

She talked about the loop of a compulsion, or obsession, which, once it took hold, repeated itself in an endless cycle; and the sufferer's attempts to avoid the obsession, or compulsion, which became all consuming.

The avoidant behaviour, making the sufferer even more anxious to stifle the impulses, by repeating the ritualistic behavior. Several patients asked what caused O.C.D.

Gabrielle explained that it was thought to be a combination of genetic and hereditary factors, chemical, structural, and functional cerebral abnormalities, and on occasion, environmental influences.

Gabrielle then asked everyone in the group, who felt comfortable enough, to talk about the reason for their hospitalization.

Jane was the first person to speak, saying she was a thirty-year-old married woman, with a young family. She spoke of the compulsions that had become overwhelming since the birth of her second child.

She described getting up at night, thirty to forty times to check that the baby was breathing.

The cleaning rituals before she could make the baby a bottle; handling the bottle of baby formula using tongs, which was awkward and time consuming. The fear that the bottle was contaminated, and pouring the milk away to start the process again. The inability to concentrate during the day because she was exhausted.

Gabrielle saw the woman sitting next to Jane, reach out, and touch her shoulder.

Robert was a teacher, also crippled by O.C.D.

His took the form of fearing he would be responsible for the death of a pedestrian, a cyclist, or another driver, caused by his failure to drive 'properly', as he described it.

When he drove past a cyclist, along the road, he turned back to make sure that no one was lying injured, because of his carelessness. He checked the newspaper, before his first class, to see that no one had been reported as being killed in a car accident, convinced that police were looking for him.

He was aware that his fears were not based on fact, nonetheless, he was compelled to repeat his rituals. In the last month, he had stopped driving, so crippling was his fear of injuring an innocent person.

He said the amount he spent weekly on taxis was astronomical, and the disorder affected his whole family.

Gabrielle took this opportunity to talk about the characteristics of people with obsessive compulsive traits. Being preoccupied with rules and details, a perfectionist, a workaholic, inflexible, a hoarder, stingy, and determined to get their own way. Very unappealing.

The group laughed at that.

Ben, an eighteen-year-old man, was eager to talk about his sexual addiction.

He said he had engaged in a relationship with his 'cousin', when he was fifteen, and she in her late twenties. He was an attractive man, tall, and well built.

Gabrielle could imagine that he looked older than his age, at fifteen.

He looked to be in his mid-twenties now. Several patients voiced their dismay at cousins, especially a fifteen-year-old, engaged in sexual behaviour. Ben responded.

"She wasn't really my cousin, it was my dad's second marriage, so we weren't related."

Robert shook his head.

"Doesn't matter, you were a child."

Ben shrugged.

"I wanted to; she was gorgeous."

"Ben, the point has been made that you were being taken advantage of. You were a child; you can't give consent to sexual behaviour with an adult when you're fifteen. It's paedophilia, child exploitation."

Gabrielle's voice was quiet, but firm.

Checking her watch, she added.

" We must leave it at that, and talk about it next time if Ben wishes."

The time had passed quickly, and Gabrielle thanked the participants.

"Take any pamphlet you wish from the bookshelf. I'll be here at the same time, every Monday, Wednesday day, and Friday afternoon".

They thanked her, smiling, and Gabrielle was glad to think that she might be able show them that they could be helped.

She resolved to use some time off duty period to write more notes which she could use in her next class. She checked the voicemail machine.

May, asking if she was able to catch up for coffee, the following day?

Daniel, with a similar request. She frowned, conflicted. She valued his friendship, he, however, had made his feelings crystal clear.

How to discourage his romantic interest, she had no idea.

She was aware that her blossoming relationship with Connor created problems with Daniel. He had been abrupt in his manner to her on one occasion, when he phoned, and she spoke briefly to him, apologizing, and explaining that Connor was with her.

Chapter Twelve

It was very apparent that the two men disliked each other.

Gabrielle, peace loving, struggled with the knowledge that she was the cause of their antipathy. On reflection, she acknowledged that the beautiful Olivia was also a substantial part of the mix.

As always, it occurred to her that, in her professional life, she could do no wrong. Her personal life was a vastly different matter.

Try as she might, she rated a two out of ten for her love life. Laughing softly, amused at her own assessment, she turned on the television, relishing the thought of a quiet evening, a solitary meal, and her favourite shows on the 'box.'

She slept well, waking refreshed, at seven o'clock. Saturday, how delightful to have Saturday off duty.

After a hasty shower, and an equally hasty breakfast, Gabrielle found a bag suitable for her various bits and pieces and made her way downstairs.

May had been busy. On the clothesline washing danced in the breeze. Gabrielle smiled at the neighbour's cat, which lay gracefully atop the brick wall dividing the properties.

May was her first port of call, and as she entered the house, on May's 'come in', she smiled at how fond she had become of this pillar of strength.

Gabrielle, ever organized, was writing their plans for the Christmas holidays, presents, festive food, off duty hours, so that she knew when, to do what.

She laughed when May said, "I wish I had some method to get my affairs in order"'

She made a mental note to buy May a diary.

Swiftly the day passed, and tasks completed, the two settled in front of the fire, trays on laps to talk and eat. Gabrielle had confided in May over her growing concern about Richard, and the Connor, Olivia disharmony.

May nodded, agreeing with Gabrielle's comment that she wanted no part of it, despite her attraction towards Connor. So the evening passed, and in bed that night she drowsily reflected that her life, apart from a few hiccups, was on track, at last.

The next weeks passed without incident. She enjoyed her work, her friendship with May, and the peace from knowing that Richard was but a fleeting thought.

Going past Connor's office, on her way home one afternoon, she was surprised to hear voices, raised in dissension. Closer, now, she recognized Olivia's voice, and it was very apparent that Olivia was weeping. Stunned, Gabrielle beat a hasty retreat, thankful to reach her car.

Driving home, she was aware that her strategy of avoiding Connor, and not responding to his phone calls or messages and the flowers delivered by courier had made little difference.

Troubled, she spent the rest of the day, fearful of a ring at the door. She listened to the phone ring, waiting until the answering machine picked up; knowing this was no way to live her life, afraid to answer the doorbell, or pick up the phone.

Reluctantly, she acknowledged, she must confront Connor. She was working a late shift the following day, and arrived at the hospital a half hour, intent on seeing Connor.

At her knock on the door, Connor called. "It's open."

Surprise visible on his face, he rose, holding out his arms to embrace her. She shook her head.

"Connor, I heard Olivia crying, as I walked past your office on the way home yesterday. I wanted to make certain that I'm not the cause of her distress."

His expression troubled, he responded.

"We spent some time together and it didn't take me long to realise she wanted a permanent commitment, she won't take 'no' for an answer."

"I've told her that at best we can be friends, however she's not willing to accept that."

"Lately, she's taken to stalking me although she says it's a coincidence that wherever I go she's not far behind."

Clearly he was troubled by Olivia's obsessive behaviour.

"She knows I feel strongly about you and she's making my life miserable."

Gabrielle sat quietly absorbing the impact of his disclosure.

"Gabrielle, you must know how I feel about you. Avoiding me isn't going to work. I've had no interest in the opposite sex since Clare died, then... you. Don't say you aren't attracted to me; we both know that's not true".

Quietly, not meeting his eyes, she glanced at her watch.

"Connor, Richard's deceit has left me wanting no personal involvement with anyone, despite my attraction to them"

Gabrielle, you can't mean that. He was a rogue."

"I won't interfere between you and Olivia. Please understand, I haven't have the emotional stability to even contemplate another relationship."

"What are you saying? You don't even want my friendship?"

She bit her lip. "Forgive me. I must go".

"Gabrielle..."

She fled, leaving the door ajar, tears filling her eyes. She realised her feelings for him, far exceeded friendship, however, she was unwilling to embark on another relationship, so soon.

Work kept her occupied until handover at 11.30pm, and wearily she made her way homeward.

Pulling into the driveway, her headlights illuminated the floral arrangement on the porch.

Her sleep that night was troubled, and by 6am the following morning she had showered and dressed, wondering what the day would bring.

Her late shift was uneventful, she was used to her charges, and they were familiar with her

The group gathered in the room set aside for patient therapy, and having made a drink from the tea trolley, sat ready to continue the work.

Gabrielle asked Ben if he had thought about the previous day's therapy, and with a frown, he said he had, could he talk about it?

Quietly, he began to speak, the group absorbed, as he told of the years from the age of thirteen to his recent eighteenth birthday.

He was in constant trouble at school because of his inability to concentrate on lessons. Flirting, sending notes to female classmates, and completely oblivious of the teacher or the lesson being taught.

His inability to hand in homework, and leaving school without graduating.

He spoke about the succession of jobs because of the ongoing inability to concentrate on the task at hand, his mind occupied with the next sexual adventure.

His parents anger at him when he was sixteen, and a neighbour's fifteen-year-old daughter became pregnant, saying Ben was the father of the baby she would not abort.

Leaving home, couch surfing, his trouble with the police when he was caught stealing food from the supermarket.

He admitted he was currently being supervised by a social worker, and that being in the hospital was the most stable environment he had experienced for many years. Several of the female patients were visibly upset at Ben's honesty. Gabrielle asked Ben how he felt about his numerous sexual encounters, over the last few years.

"I hate myself; I don't know why I chase skirt. Once I've had sex, I can't get away quick enough. I shower every time I have sex, six and seven times a day."

Then an hour later I'm out looking for another bird".

Someone in the group asked. "Are you saying you had sex with different women six or seven times a day?"

Ben nodded. "Sometimes more…"

Gabrielle said quietly. "That is the nature of sexual obsessive-compulsive behaviour."

"Ben has just demonstrated how obsessive-compulsive disorder ruins lives, not that anyone in the group fails to understand the grip it has on daily lives."

"Next, if no one else wishes to speak, we'll talk about treatment options, and the support available, so that sufferers of O.C.D. can live a life, not entirely stress free, but certainly not the unhappy life you all live now.

"If anyone wants a tea, or toilet break, now's a good time, we've another hour before we finish this afternoon. Several members left the room, and Gabrielle took the opportunity to look at her notes. Once settled, she asked, "has anyone had therapy thus far?"

No one had, although Robert had sought help from his family doctor, who was at a loss to offer advice.

Robert said. "He must have thought I was mad; he's been our doctor since I was a child, but I had no one else to turn to."

"When I said I kept going back to check that I hadn't knocked someone down, he just shook his head, and didn't say a thing. I told my wife I was seeing him once a week, but I wasn't."

"My wife said I didn't get help, we'd have to separate, she was tired of it."

"I've got two small kids, I can't lose them because of this rotten obsession."

There were murmurs of assent, and several other members nodded in agreement.

"Let's talk about help then. At the moment, group therapy and talking about obsessions, and being compelled to repeat certain actions, or behaviors, is ongoing for each of you."

"Being able to discuss anything without ridicule, disgust, or disagreement in a group setting is vital".

"We've talked about cognitive behavioural therapy, of confronting your fears, not avoiding that which you fear, and not giving in to rituals. So called exposure therapy, exposing yourself to your fears and staying on course, as it were."

"Recently, certain medications have proved very successful in the treatment of O.C.D."

"Each of you will have outpatient care when you leave the hospital, and your doctor will prescribe any medication, including anti-depressants, that are best suited to you."

"We've spoken about side effects, and you know your G.P is competent to treat any problems regarding medication."

"Lastly, we've talked about yoga, aromatherapy, meditation, and relaxation, you've heard the tapes and been shown the techniques, and you know these are an ongoing support."

Karen, a young woman who never spoke in the group, surprised Gabrielle by saying hesitantly.

"I was reading about Howard Hughes, the American billionaire. I wondered if you could tell the group about him?"

"Certainly, although you've read his story, would you like to tell the group?".

The young woman shook her head, and Gabrielle smiled at her.

"As Karen says, Hughes was an American billionaire, brilliant, innovative, and complex. He was an industrialist who made his fortune from making films and designing and building planes."

"He owned hotels and casinos in Las Vegas, and the Howard Hughes Medical Institute, in Miami, Florida. "I think there's mention of designing a brassiere for the actress Jane Russell, whether that's fact, I don't know.

Also, the character of Iron Man was based on Hughes. He was renowned for making the classic film, 'Hell's Angels'.""

"Hughes had a very close relationship with his overprotective mother, who focused her attention on her only child.

She was a powerful and dominant force in his life, and most likely instilled a fear of germs in him at a very early age. She died, when he was sixteen, and two years later his father died, making him an orphan."

"His response to this was to become a very strong willed, dominant character, allowing no one to tell him how to live his life. Control, Hughes life was all about controlling his world."

"He was also renowned for working forty hours at a stretch, day or night, with an occasional break to eat a can of beans or a sandwich. So, clearly indicating his eccentricities."

"His relationship with film stars and socialites was legendary. He was the man who brought a bit player, Arlene Carpenter, later called Jean Harlow, to the public's attention."

"Would anyone like to comment on what you've heard so far?"

Karen said, "He was the poster child for total control.?"
Gabrielle nodded.

"All forecasting the eventual descent into madness, not to put too fine a point on it."

The group were fascinated.

Robert asked. "What happened to him? I've never heard of him before. I'm going to get any books or whatever I can, so I can read about him. He makes my O.C.D. look mild by comparison."

Everyone laughed.

Gabrielle said, "Hughes crashed a plane, suffered serious burns and injuries, and became addicted to narcotics to manage the pain. "

"He recovered, and his life went on in much the same manner. He was shy, yet he was known as a ladies' man. "

"He dated Marilyn Monroe, and would have dated Elizabeth Taylor, however she refused."

Again, the group laughed.

"Hughes began exhibiting obvious signs of O.C.D. in his early twenties, compulsive hand washing, checking, and re checking work, even down to wanting a particular cloud formation in his plane films".

"All indications of extreme O.C.D, with underlying phobic tendencies. It was during this period that his extreme phobia of germs surfaced."
" He'd moved into a bungalow at the Beverly Hills hotel, and later, a suite in some other hotel."

" Karen would know which hotel; it escapes me at the moment. Gradually over the years, his life became a spiral of drug dependency, and compulsive cleansing rituals of objects he or his carers touched."

"He stopped showering or bathing, wouldn't have his hair, his fingernails or his toenails cut. He even collected his bodily waste in jars, so intense and out of control was his obsession"

"His carers, all men, were made to follow a handbook of rules regarding their interactions with him."
" His drug addiction controlled his life, and when he died he weighed around seventy pounds."

"One of, if not the, richest men in America dying like a pauper. It was said that he was taken advantage of financially by certain carers."

"Well, no doubt after that, you're all looking forward to a cup of coffee, so we'll finish for today."

"I'd like to say, 'good work' to all of you, I know it's confronting to talk about."

"Oh, just a thought, romantic love is biologically indistinguishable from a severe obsessive-compulsive disorder."

They all laughed, although it was apparent that hearing about Howard Hughes tragic life had given them food for thought. As usual, each person in the group thanked her, smiling, and as they made for the door, talking and laughing.

So very different, Gabrielle thought, from these same people in the first few days of group therapy. She felt a quiet glow of satisfaction, a feeling of pleasure that she had been instrumental in helping them live a more calm and peaceful existence.

 It was what she was born to do. She smiled, thinking that she was glad her thoughts weren't displayed in a bubble above her head the way certain cartoon characters were.

The rest of the shift passed without incident, and soon she was heading home, tired but content.

She slept until eight a.m. the following day and was up and showered when May arrived at the house. She smiled at Gabrielle.

"I've had breakfast, but I wouldn't mind a cup of coffee."

May settled herself in front of the log fire while Gabrielle filled the jug.

"How's the group therapy going?"

"May, they're all such decent people, so willing to do whatever it takes to improve their lives."

Talking, and drinking their coffee, they made plans for Christmas. May knew Gabrielle had volunteered to work an early shift on Christmas morning, which suited her. She could put the finishing touches to the midday Christmas dinner. May's son and both grandchildren would visit for the day. They had shopped for food and gifts at the Central market, and Gabrielle had her presents wrapped and ready.

Christmas eve was on Friday, then Gabrielle had the weekend off duty until the following Monday afternoon. On Christmas

Eve, Gabrielle spent time with the patients deemed too unwell to be at home on Christmas day.

There were fewer patients to care for and no group therapy, so the nurses concentrating on making the ward as cheerful as possible. Staff and patients hung decorations and trimmed the Christmas tree. Presents for all were underneath the tree, and the mood was one of cheer.

By ten p.m. all the patients were in bed. The ward was darkened, and Gabrielle was sitting in the office writing the report.

 On the way home that night, she thought about her first Christmas in Australia It was December, hot and humid, and so different from the snow and ice that her parents would be experiencing.

She was awake and ready to leave the house by six thirty on Christmas morning. On the drive to the Q.E.H., she was amused to see cars gaily decorated with balloons, holly, and mistletoe, something she had never seen in England.

Chapter Thirteen

She was early, and made her way to the canteen for a cup of coffee, hoping to see Jo before the two went on duty. Jo was seated near the door, beckoning her over.

Jo had been invited to spend the day with May, Gabrielle, and the family, and they arranged to meet in the car park at three fifteen. The ward was bright with coloured decorations, and carols played quietly in the background.

Patients moved around the ward preparing afternoon tea to which their family were invited, an age-old tradition.

The nurses had bought small presents, bath crystals, several diaries, chocolates, and packs of different coloured pens for the patients.

The morning passed quickly, with medication the only break in the ongoing festivities. Board games, charades, and, eventually, Christmas dinner, which was served by the nursing staff. Crackers were pulled, and hats decorated blonde, brunette, and red heads.

Soon enough it was time for the change of shift, and Gabrielle made her way to the car park, where Jo was waiting. Talking and laughing, they drove to May's house.

Several cars were parked in the oval driveway, and together the two made their way to the house.

The sound of children's laughter, a deep male voice, and less audible, May, also laughing, rang clearly from outside.

They were greeted by May, and, seated in the lounge room, Jo told May and the family of their morning, while the children played with their presents.

Both nurses had apologized for keeping the family from Christmas lunch, Tom, May's son laughed. "Mum always makes such a big breakfast; we hardly have room for lunch."

Caroline, Tom's wife, smiled.

"I'm in awe of nursing and medical staff, working when everyone else is at home enjoying the day."

Gabrielle looked at Jo, and they both laughed..

" Jo and I enjoy working on Christmas Day."

May and Caroline busied themselves in the kitchen, and soon they were sitting down to the lavish meal.

Replete, Tom and Caroline put dishes in the dish washer, and they all moved back to the lounge to exchange presents.

Both children sat watching a video, while the adults talked and reminisced about Christmases past. Jo was on early duty the following day, so they thanked the family, and wished them a safe trip home. Gabrielle told May she would call her on Boxing Day.

She knew Jo was meeting friends for a night out, so she said farewell and drove home. It was cold, and the streets were deserted. She relished the thought of a quiet evening in front of the fire watching television.

As she neared the house she became aware that Connor's car was parked outside in the road, and by the time she had garaged her car, he was at the front door.

Slowly she walked towards him, surprised by the depth of her attraction towards him. He was unsure of his greeting, searching her face for a cue.

"Gabrielle, merry Christmas, how was your day?"

She unlocked the door, standing aside to let him pass. Uncertain, he remained where he was.

"Connor, it's been a long day. Do you want to come in or not?"

She entered the hall, with mixed feelings about having him in the house.

"Will you have a cup of coffee, or a drink?"

"Nothing, thank you. Gabrielle, you must know I've been miserable about our lack of contact, I've missed you, more than you know."

" If I've said something wrong, hurt you, been unfeeling, can't we sort it out?"

"Connor, I can't be any clearer in my resolve not to come between you and Olivia. I don't need to repeat that. If you don't want a drink, I'm tired and I'm going to bed."

Connor said nothing, but held his arms out, beseeching. Gabrielle bit her lip, aware that Connor had no idea of her feelings for him.

"What can I do, I can't believe this is what you want?"

"Connor, I don't want to have any conversation about you, me, or Olivia now."

"Tomorrow, then, let me take you to dinner."

"I'm busy tomorrow, then I'm working, I really don't have time."

She turned away, stricken by the pain in his face.

"Please, Gabrielle, if only you knew how that makes me feel. However, since I'm clearly wasting your time, I'll go."

Locking the door, and stoking the fire, she made her way to bed, biting her lip to keep from shedding the tears so near to the surface. She would redouble her efforts to find a job where she wouldn't cross paths with Connor on a daily basis.

The following day she was occupied, taking down decorations, and attending to the patients' needs. Over the following week, she saw Connor several times, but avoided contact with him. It occurred to her that working as an Agency R/n would offer respite from what had become a difficult situation. She phoned a local Agency and was given an appointment for the following morning.

The ward was gradually filling after the Christmas break, and at six p.m. she made her way to the canteen, smiling as she spotted Jo at a nearby table. Jo greeted her with a wide smile.

"I've been hoping you'd get the same meal break as me. How've you been doing?"

"Hi, gradually recovering after Christmas."

Talking and laughing, enjoying each other's company, the meal break was soon over, and she made her way back to the ward refreshed.

"Sister, Dr Quinlan left this for you".

Gabrielle took the envelope held out to her, aware of curiosity in Sister Henman's eyes.

Smiling her thanks, she put the envelope in her pocket. She was off duty the following day, looking forward to seeing May. They had planned to have lunch and see a film.

It took but a few minutes to shower, dress, and make her way to May's house. May, as always, was finishing some last minute chores.

"Take a seat, I won't be a moment".

Gabrielle reached for her bag, remembering Connor's letter. Her face paled as she read the brief message.

"I'm ready, are you.... Gabrielle, what is it?"

May was alarmed by her friend's pallor, aware that it was associated with the letter on the table.

Wordlessly, Gabrielle pushed the letter across to her, watching May's expression change as she read the few words on the page.

Oh Gabrielle, I'm so sorry."

"Connor said she was behaving irrationally, but to do that, it's unthinkable."

May was on her feet, filling the jug, putting out mugs.

" Let's have a cup of tea, collect our thoughts."

Despite her distress, Gabrielle laughed.

"May, why do we always have a cup of tea when we've had

disturbing news?"

May laughed too, albeit with little humour.

"It's what we Aussies do. Where is she?"

"Grange, it's a private hospital Connor has patients at."

"Connor won't look after her will he?"

Gabrielle shook her head.

"No, she'll be treated by another psychologist"

"It's not ethical to treat a patient one has had a relationship with."

"As he says in the letter, it was intended to force him into making a commitment to her rather than a genuine attempt to end her life."

May brought the tray to the table and filled the mugs from the teapot.

Quietly, both women sat, pondering the fact that Olivia had attempted suicide by taking an overdose of barbiturates, however halfhearted the attempt.

Gabrielle wondered how Connor was dealing with the news, knowing that he was the reason for Olivia's misery, and that she too was indirectly involved.

"May, you realise I can't stay here; it's made that impossible."

"Gabrielle, you're not at fault, there's no reason for you to leave."

" Connor mustn't know how I feel. Before I met him Olivia was very much a part of his life. I imagine they would have married eventually."

"It makes me realise that working so close to him and seeing him every day is impossible. I love him, May, he's everything Richard isn't"

"I'm so sorry, I'd give anything to make you stay, however I must admit I can understand how difficult that would make life for you."

So it was with sadness at leaving May, her work, and the home she had grown fond of, that Gabrielle gave her notice, and contacted the real estate agent.

To say he was surprised was an understatement. An unforeseen family emergency, Gabrielle explained, disliking the untruth but with no other option

Packing her personal possessions took minutes, and with a last look at the little house she had called home for such a brief time, she locked the front door.

The keys had been left by arrangement with May.

Sad at what she was doing, Gabrielle departed for fresh fields.

She had phoned her parents the previous evening with the news that she had decided to see Australia by applying for jobs as an Agency R/n.

No need to worry them about the reason for her decision. They were happy for her. 'Send us postcards, and phone, stay safe, we love you', was their response.

The appointment with the nursing Agency was on the following morning, and she had no difficulty finding her way to the office. The Agency owner, Rebecca, was pleased to add a triple certificate R/n to her workforce.

Was Gabrielle interested in working in the small town of Covell, on the Eyre Peninsula? Alice Springs?

After a few questions about Covell, Gabrielle agreed that Covell sounded delightful. Rebecca assured Gabrielle that she would make a weekly call to ascertain that Gabrielle was content at Covell.

Gabrielle had learned that Covell was situated on the Eyre Peninsula, bordered by the Great Australian Bight, the Gawler Ranges, and Spencer Gulf.

Eyre Peninsula was named after explorer, Edward John Eyre, who set foot there in the year 1839. Looking at the map, Gabrielle learned it was a 636.5 kilometre drive from Adelaide to Covell, necessitating an overnight stay somewhere.

Intent on an early start the next day, she started preparing.

The car was serviced, she had her hair cut, and visited a small boutique for some suitable beachside clothes. Finally, she booked into a small hotel to spend the night.

The dining room menu was extensive; however, she chose a light meal, and, weary after a long day, made her way to her room.

She had a quick shower the following morning, then dressed in slacks and a long-sleeved blouse, and made her way down to the dining room.

The chef had prepared a packed lunch for the long drive, and having paid her account, she took the lift down to the garage to begin the trip to Covell.

The day was fine, the sky blue, and leaving the city behind, she took to the open road without a problem.

She enjoyed driving, listening to classical music on the radio and contemplating the adventure of the next however many months.

Wistfully, she thought of the brief note she had left for Connor, knowing he would be sad that she was no longer within arm's reach.

She knew Olivia had been discharged from hospital and would receive psychological support out in the community.

The countryside was beautiful, green and ever changing. Endless pastures with herds of Jersey cows grazing, fields of rapeseed, and sheep cropping the grass.

She took several rest stops along the way, stretching, and saying a quiet 'thank you' to the chef, for her small lunch basket. She made good time, and in midafternoon she entered the small township of Covell.

The area, with its fishing, oyster port, and holiday resort, was surprisingly quiet. Probably holidaymakers were at the beach or exploring the many activities on offer.

Covell hospital would be by far the smallest Gabrielle had ever worked at.

She parked the car and entered the main entrance. It was a twenty-bed facility, catering for acute and aged care patients, with a small accident and emergency department and operating theatre.

She knew that patients in need of specialised care were transferred to Whyalla, or any one of the Adelaide hospitals.

Giving her name at reception, she was told that a staff member would be available to take her to the nurses' quarters.

A short wait until a young woman in the white uniform and white shoes so familiar to her appeared, smiling a welcome. "Good trip?"

Gabrielle returned the smile.

"Thank you, yes, I enjoyed it. "

Talking, they made their way to the cottage, which housed live-in staff.

Kathryn filled in the blanks about the nursing Director, and the doctor, who was the only medical person available in the area, and finally, expressed her gratitude that a triple certificate R/n would be on staff.

Gabrielle was intrigued by the admission.

" Sounds like there've been difficulties in attracting staff to the hospital?'

Kathryn laughed. "You could say that, not everyone with your qualifications wants to work in a small country hospital, however beautiful the location."

Gabrielle smiled. "Since I'm from London, this is heaven on earth."

"I'll let you settle in, then take you to nursing admin."

Gabrielle thanked the young woman, remarking,

"Kathryn, such a pretty name."

Kathryn grinned. "You're going to fit right in."

A brief time later, the two young women entered nursing admin.

"I'll come back, when you're ready, Jan, (the secretary,) will let me know."

Knocking on the door, Gabrielle was bid enter. The nursing Director greeted her, motioning her to a chair.

"Miss Graham, I'm so happy to welcome you to our small community".

"Thank you, Miss Ryan".

" Since you're accredited in three fields of nursing, I hope you don't object to being on call for mid and general. We don't have much call for nursing patients with psychiatric disorders."

"Whatever is necessary, Miss Ryan, I enjoy both."

"Well, then, we'll see you on duty tomorrow. I'll start you in the general ward, then, if there's an R/n in charge, you can discuss off duty hours with her. I hope we let you learn the ropes before you're in charge.

"Thank you, I'm well able to adapt."

"Looking at your qualifications my dear, I have no doubt of that."

Gabrielle was relieved, glad that she was welcomed into the small hospital.

The following morning, she asked the clerk in nursing admin, where she was rostered on duty.

She was told she would work on the medical, surgical, paediatric, and orthopaedic wards, all housed in one small area, and comprising twenty patients.

Midwifery, Casualty, and theatre had nursing staff rostered separately to those areas. At the nurses station, she was greeted by the night duty R/n, Staff nurse Clark.

"Good morning Sister, and welcome, I know you'll be keen to get started."

Gabrielle smiled. "Good morning, yes, I'm looking forward to it. I hope you had a quiet night?"

"No dramas, so your first day should be the same, it'll give you time to catch up with what's happening".

Gabrielle took notes and asked a few questions, then having checked the D.D.A. Dangerous Drug Act drugs, morphine, Pethidine, and the premed phials, and ensured a correct count, the staff nurse left the ward. Gabrielle introduced herself to her staff nurse, and the enrolled nurses. She would oversee all staff in Lincoln, the name all the general wards were grouped under.

Chapter Fourteen

With her staff nurse, Gabrielle moved from one room to another, introducing herself and asking each patient something about the reason they were in the hospital.

Staff nurse Clark was thorough in sharing each patient's medical history with Gabrielle. By the time they reached the end room it was morning tea break, and Gabrielle returned to the office.

Clark had mentioned that she and Staff nurse Morgan, whom Gabrielle had yet to meet, worked opposite shifts. Then, having collected her bag, Clark and the two e/ns went off duty.

By the end of her shift, Gabrielle knew all she needed to know about those in her care.

She considered she was fortunate with her staff. Clark, and all the e/ns were industrious and knowledgeable about the patients.

The following day, Gabrielle worked a late shift. She had written the staff off duty roster the previous day, ensuring each shift was covered by an R/n, and two e/n's.

The evening shift was uneventful. Two children on the children's ward, having t's and a's, medical lingo for tonsillectomy and adenoidectomy. A five-year-old, with Cystic Fibrosis, an autoimmune disease, and a toddler with ectopic dermatitis.

Admission days were Monday, and Wednesday, for t's and a's. The child with C.F., and the toddler remained in the ward until their condition improved, since both ailments were lifelong conditions.

In the male ward were five adults suffering different illnesses, which kept staff busy.

In the next ward, one man with diabetes, one with C.O.P.D, chronic obstructive airways disease, one obese man for weight control regulation, prior to bariatric surgery, and two middle aged men, one with a chest infection, the other with congestive cardiac failure.

Another six bedded ward housed young men, all with various fractures sustained in motorbike accidents, roller blading, and diving from a diving board.

In the four bedded female ward, there were patients for three different surgical procedures. tubal ligation, hysterectomy, and varicose vein surgery, and one young woman with cystitis.

Twenty two patients in all

No conditions Gabrielle hadn't seen in previous jobs. So, the week passed quickly.

Off duty. Gabrielle walked around the small town, bought several fiction novels, explored the beach, and was glad she had decided to join the Agency.

As Gabrielle expected, no two days were the same. Patients went home, cured, or, at least, improved, and others took their place. Of all the patients, two proved to be long term.

Mr. Bartlett, with airways disease, and Mr. Kaye, who suffered from congestive cardiac disease, both men needing continuous oxygen.

Gabrielle enjoyed working with all the nursing staff, and they with her.

She learned, through a chance remark, that she was valued, because she 'pulled her weight'; unlike other agency R'n's, who preferred to remain in the office, leaving bed making and other work to the hospital staff.

Gabrielle helped make beds, gave medications, and talked to patients, whilst she gave blanket baths, and generally,' mucked in,' and this differentiated her from other Agency staff. A knock on the door made her pause.

"Come in, Nurse Wilson."

Nurse Wilson, recently qualified, was very pale, and Gabrielle stood, wondering if the girl was ill.

" Sister, I can't get Mr. Kaye's blood pressure."

Gabrielle was on her feet immediately, and seconds later at the man's side. Given that Mr. Kaye had a cardiac disorder, Gabrielle surmised he had suffered a cardiac arrest. She smiled at Wilson.

"He didn't suffer, he probably had no idea of what was happening."

"Sister, shall I get the mortuary pack?"

"Please, I'll let Dr Myers know."

Leaving a message for Dr Myers, Gabrielle returned to the ward, where Wilson was washing the dead man's face.

"I'm glad Mr. Bartlett's not back until tomorrow".

Wilson nodded.

"Yes, it would have upset him, they're mates."

Quietly, they worked, until Mr. Kaye was ready for a mortuary gown.

"I'll make a quick round, will you put the kettle on, if it's quiet, we'll have a cup of coffee."

All was quiet, and Gabrielle joined Wilson in the kitchen.

"It's as well ..."

The phone rang, startling them both. Gabrielle listened, as Dr Myers spoke.

"…. he came off his motorbike, I know we don't have a spare bed, but I'll be in early tomorrow, see who's ready for discharge."

The only bed available was in the room where Mr. Kaye lay at peace. Nurse Wilson had joined Gabrielle in the office.

"Sister, I've made a pot of coffee."

Gabrielle shook her head.

" No time, we've an admission, you'll probably know him, a local lad, according to Dr. Myers".

"Sister, we don't have a bed."

"Which means Mr. Kaye will have to be moved into the garage."

Swiftly, Mr. Kaye was moved onto a gurney, both nurses thankful the man was small, and thin.

Armed with umbrellas, and with the gurney covered by a tarpaulin, Gabrielle, and Wilson, both wearing Macintoshes, made certain the corridor was clear.

The rain was torrential. Hurrying, Gabrielle guided the gurney, the path to the garage lit by Wilsons' torch. Wilson, wet, and with shaky hands, put the key into the lock. Several seconds passed as Wilson tried to unlock the garage door.

"Sister, the key won't turn, there's…."

With a loud crack, the key broke off in the lock. Wilson was horrified, giving vent to her feelings.

"Jesus, Mary, and Joseph…"

Wilson's Irish nationality well to the fore.

Gabrielle, eyes blurred by rain, was aware that the young woman was mortified.

"Nurse Wilson, let's not panic, where're the spare keys kept?"

"There's no spare key."

"There must be some way of getting the door open, surely?"

"Oh Sister, it's my feck….it's my fault, I'm so sorry."

"Nurse Wilson, who's the gardener, or the handyman; who does the gardening or whatever's needed at the hospital?"

Wilson shook her head.

"Miss Ryan gets someone in when its necessary."

" It's necessary, is there someone I can call?"

Weeping now, Wilson shook her soaking head, having dropped the umbrella in her panic.

To her dismay, Gabrielle felt a bubble of laughter in her throat. This was a disastrous situation.

Mr. Kaye, still dry under the tarpaulin, neither knew nor cared of the difficulties experienced by his previous saviours.

Gabrielle, who was also soaked, and shivering, was aware of the humour in the situation, and couldn't help but laugh.

Nurse Wilson, teeth chattering, stared at her senior, then she too began to laugh.

Soaked, and shivering, both women vented their feelings, before Gabrielle remembered the admission.

"Is there nowhere we can put Mr. Kaye?"

For some reason, known only to Wilson, the question caused another eruption of mirth.

Realising the girl was close to hysteria, Gabrielle said sharply.

"Wilson, pull yourself together, the admission will be here before we know where we are."

"Sorry Sister, I've never seen a dead person before.

"Then Mr. Kaye will have to stay here."

This seemed to be the only solution, so, leaving Mr. Kaye to brave the elements, or at least, the gurney, and ensuring the tarpaulin could not be dislodged by the howling wind, they made their way back to the hospital.

They took turns going to their rooms to put on a dry uniform, and as Gabrielle made her way back to the hospital, the small vehicle used to transport patients arrived at the front door.

Gabrielle accompanied the stretcher to the recently vacated room. The young man on the gurney smelt strongly of alcohol, and appeared to be in a jovial mood.

He was swiftly transferred to the bed, asleep now and snoring loudly, whilst his vital signs were recorded.

Wilson began undressing him, and Gabrielle had a brief conversation with the driver before joining Nurse Wilson. As they dressed him in a gown, Dr Myers entered the room.

"Ah, Sister, he's in good hands, I've already examined him. He's got a nasty injury. He managed to get one of the bike's handlebars in his rectum."

"Fortunately it didn't perforate anything, Of course, he's drunk as a skunk, so he's feeling no pain. I've written him up for morphine and antibiotics, and I'll check in on him tomorrow. Sorry about an admission at this hour."

"Now, where's Mr. Kaye?"

With a start, Gabrielle remembered where Mr. Kaye was. Leaving Nurse Wilson, Gabrielle made her way to the office.

Eyebrows raised, Dr Myers asked, "a problem?"

"You could say that".

As Gabrielle explained the 'problem', Myers, as first frowning, burst into laughter and much relieved Gabrielle joined him, describing Nurse Wilson's lapse into Irish mode.

Dr Myer's laughed heartily at this.

"Poor young woman, her first experience of death, pouring with rain, and she makes a hash of it, hardly surprising. Perhaps I should have a quick word with her to make sure she's alright."

"Would you, Doctor, she was so upset."

Myers smiled at the beautiful young woman, wondering again, why a woman with such striking looks would want to be a nurse, and smiling at such a politically incorrect observation.

Gabrielle looked at the vital signs, recorded by Wilson. All within normal limits. His colour was good, and he was, as Nurse Wilson often said, 'Away with the fairies.'

Leaving the overhead light on, Gabrielle walked into the office. Nurse Wilson, smiling now, asked. "Sister, will I put the jug on?"

"Have your break now, while its quiet."

Smiling at Dr. Myers, she asked, "Will you have a cup of coffee?"

"Love one, white, no sugar."

She busied herself in the kitchen, smiling again, when Myers said, "A real baptism by fire, since you came to Oz."

Laughing, she nodded, "You could say that. I've never worked in a country hospital before, so very different from city hospitals".

"Worse, or not too bad?"

"I've enjoyed it tremendously, apart from leaving poor Mr. Kaye out in a storm."

"Not your fault, my dear, and no reason why anyone should know. Michael will be out for the count for a few hours, so Mr. Kaye can come back here."

"Thank you, I couldn't think of where to put him."

"All's well that ends well, I'll see you in a few hours, since its already four o'clock."

"Leave the mug Doctor, I'll put it in the dishwasher."

Smiling at her, Myers left, thinking that the man fortunate enough to secure this remarkable young woman's affections was blessed indeed.

Meanwhile, starting at young Michael's room, Gabrielle walked around the rooms, thankful that all the patients slept. Back in the office, she commenced writing the report, noting that all patients had appeared to sleep well.

She added Michael's name to the T.P.R. book. His observations would be taken two hourly now, until his medical status could be assessed when he regained consciousness, after the initial intravenous morphine. Dr. Myers had not deemed it necessary to put a cannula into a wrist vein, given the boy's stable observations.

Any analgesic needed could be given orally.

At seven am, the day duty nurses appeared, and Gabrielle wished Nurse Wilson a restful sleep, and gave the report, adding that Michael had been given a quarter of morphine intramuscularly at six thirty am, to be given four hourly, p. r. n., Pro Re Nata, Latin for 'as required'.

His observations, stable, were now being recorded four hourly, no urine specimen had been obtained, and he remained asleep, thankfully, since Mr. Kaye was in the bed next to him. Dr Myers would be in shortly to discharge someone and free up a bed.

She said, given that Michael had not had fluids since prior to admission, an intravenous infusion trolley was ready in the room, should he need I.v fluids.

Lastly, she reported that the key to the garage had broken in the lock, could Clark see that the lock was replaced. Clark raised her eyebrows but refrained from comment.

Staff nurse Clark signed the D.D.A book, and, Gabrielle, tired, but thankful the night was over, left the ward. The rain had stopped, and the sky was blue. Gabrielle changed quickly into civvies and made her way to the beach.

Seagulls wheeled overhead, and slowly she made her way over the wet sand, stopping to pick up shells.

Thinking of the night, she laughed softly, recalling the look on Wilson's face as the key broke in the lock. She would make it a priority to ensure that the lock was changed, and several keys left in the office, although she doubted such a thing could happen twice.

Weary now, she returned to the hospital, happy that the small Nurses home was quiet, and she would sleep peacefully, thinking that no two duties were the same.

That evening, Staff nurse Carroll was on duty.

Much had changed, several patients discharged, Mr. Bartlett readmitted for 'maintenance', another man for gastric ulcer investigation, and… Michael.

Chapter Fifteen

Michael, this evening, was very different from Michael of the early hours of the morning.

Pale, and nauseous, despite Maxolon, an anti-emetic being given earlier, he held a vomit bowl, barely acknowledging her.

"Not feeling too good?"

Gabrielle took his wrist, feeling for the radial pulse. Elevated, however, considering his pallor and nausea, unsurprising.

She noted his pulse on the observation chart, and checked the intravenous, running at a steady pace.

His urinary drainage bag, containing at least a hundred mls of blood-stained urine, told its own story, and with a gentle pat on his shoulder, Gabrielle returned to the office.

Reading his notes she saw that he had sustained trauma to the kidneys, the rectal injury not considered to be severe.

With bed rest, careful monitoring of fluid intake and output, antibiotics, and pain relief, he should make a full recovery.

Hopefully, he would also learn that alcohol, and motorbikes or fast cars were not a good combination.

The following day, a young woman, possibly in the second trimester of pregnancy was admitted. She said she had received no antenatal care, and only visited the GP that morning because she felt unwell.

This was her first pregnancy, and she was unsure of the father. Urine and blood samples were taken by Gabrielle, who asked an E/n to test the urine and commence the usual charts.

The young woman sat in bed, awaiting the doctor's visit.

Gabrielle noted that Anne had an elevated blood pressure, indicating early onset gestational hypertension, high blood pressure associated with pregnancy.

The E/n returning to the room, wrote the urinalysis on the chart, handing it to Gabrielle.

She was not surprised to see that the urine contained an excessive amount of protein in the sample. She was aware that the severe headaches, visual disturbance, shortness of breath, upper abdominal pain, nausea, and a decreased urine output, which Anne described, were all markers for pre-eclampsia.

Anne's face was swollen, as were her ankles.

The goal would be to manage the condition so that the due date of delivery would be as close as possible. Bed rest was essential, anti-convulsant drugs and medication to treat hypertension were also on her medication chart, should they become necessary.

Corticosteroids would also be given to help the baby's lungs to develop. The doctor's brief examination confirmed Gabrielle's suspicions.

Anne was in the early stages of pre-eclampsia. Fortunately, with rest and medication, Anne's pregnancy would continue without further complications.

Likewise, Michael, who was now getting up during the day, and moving freely around the hospital. Both children with chronic illnesses had been discharged, as had Mr. Bartlett, for Outpatient follow-up.

The next day was an admission day was an admission day. The usual conditions, one man for tonsillectomy, one for orchiectomy, removal of a testicle, for a malignant tumour.

Two female patients for tubal ligation, two toddlers with croup, and several elderly patients, awaiting placement in nursing homes. Last a young woman with a diagnosis of Systemic Lupus Erythematosus.

Gabrielle had never nursed a patient with Lupus, although she had studied the disease, and was familiar with it in theory. She knew it was one of a group of so-called autoimmune disorders, where the body attacks its own healthy tissue in all parts of the body.

Lupus was characterized by multisystem inflammation, and the production of antibodies, causing damage to the skin, blood cells, joints, and brain. A truly frightening disease. Several patients were moved into different rooms, to free up a single room. Gabrielle was off duty that day, when the patient was transferred to the Royal Adelaide hospital, which didn't surprise her.

The hospital was too small, with insufficient facilities to care for critically ill patients.

So her last week at Covell passed uneventfully, and it was with regret that she farewelled the staff she had enjoyed working with.

On her last day, the staff and patients had held a small afternoon tea in her honour, genuinely sorry that this knowledgeable, kind, industrious R/n was leaving.

She was amused, on opening her suitcases, to see that confetti decorated the contents. Once again, she was on the move, wondering how long it would be before Agency nursing lost its appeal.

The letter from May that week had little to add to letters sent in previous weeks. May always ended her letters by asking Gabrielle when she would be home.

Daniel, too, wrote weekly. The house had been sold for an excellent price, they were busy at work, and as always, he missed her, when would she be home?

Unlike May, Daniel had no idea that Gabrielle leaving so precipitately was a direct result of her involvement with Connor, and Olivia's suicide attempt.

Indeed, Daniel knew nothing about Gabrielle's budding relationship with Connor.

Gabrielle missed Connor, his voice, the touch of his hand, the smile which lit his eyes, the way his voice grew husky when he said her name.

She admired his honesty and compassion, his willingness to take up arms for a cause he believed in.

He was the man she wanted in her life, although she had been unaware of it.

She relived their kiss, the feel of his body as he held her close, knowing that she was safe in his arms.

Unwittingly she had fallen in love with Connor, her feelings for him so different from how she had felt about Richard. Her relationship with Richard had been shallow, she realised now.

Richard was driven by his passion for material possessions, the desire to impress with the best that money could buy.

She believed her simplicity, her very naivete, had at first attracted him, so used was he to sophisticated worldly women. The attraction quickly palled when his efforts to 'educate 'her had proved unsuccessful.

She was very aware that the union would have been disastrous, given the difference in their moral principles. She mused on her life since she had arrived in Australia.

Always, before she started a road trip she made sure her cassettes were readily available.

The car had recently been fitted with new tyres and there was a good supply of petrol on board.

She was adept at changing a tyre should the need arise. Two years earlier, planning for her trip to Australia she had undertaken a course on car maintenance.

She had a good knowledge of problems in the event that she was 'out in Whoop, Whoop,' Australian slang for the middle of nowhere and ran into problems with the car.

She had started her journey early that morning and made good time to the town of Point Lowly, a distance of eighty- nine kilometres from Port Augusta.

The one hour drive was easily accomplished, and she entered the town making for the Tourist Centre.

Armed with a handful of brochures, she headed for the beach and the boats gathered on the foreshore, in the area where cuttlefish gathered to spawn.

She knew a favourite pursuit for visitors was to see giant cuttlefish from the safety of a glass bottomed boat. Although it was a sunny day, it was cold, being winter, and she was glad that she was warmly clad.

Reading the brochure, she learned that the cuttlefish arrived in Spencer Gulf in May each year to breed, and that the beautiful cephalopods, once endangered by commercial fishing, were now a protected species.

In 2013, these huge creatures numbered eight thousand only, until, recognized as endangered, the Government banned fishing and by 2019, some two hundred thousand cuttlefish congregated in the cold waters of Point Lowly, Spencer Gulf, to breed.

They were acknowledged as the largest cuttlefish in the world, reaching a total length of almost one metre and weighing up to five kilograms when eighteen months old.

Their colour changing skin cells, called chromatophores, enabled the cephalopods to change colour, making it easy to blend into their environment.

They were curious creatures, and moved by crawling, swimming, and propelling themselves through the water if something piqued their interest.

She watched mesmerized, as, only four metres below the boat, two large males were engaged in a nonviolent confrontation, each changing colour, in a spectacular neon sign colour change, to attract the attention of the smaller females.

After mating with a male partner, the female deposited her fertilized eggs under the rocks where they hatched.

The guide told the boats occupants that the cuttlefish do not eat during the mating period, becoming weaker and weaker, and metabolizing their own flesh, until, mating over, both male and female died.

She had witnessed for herself that it was also possible to dive, and get to within an arm's length of them, so engrossed were they in the mating ritual.

Gabrielle, ever the wildlife warrior, rejoiced that they were no longer seen as prey, although, as the wildlife guide explained, many species of flora and fauna had been lost to predation over the years.

It was exciting to snorkel with the cuttlefish, however the water was icy, so she contented herself with taking photos and learning about them from the knowledgeable wildlife guide.

Leaving the boat, thoroughly chilled by now, she stopped for coffee from her flask, before driving to Port Augusta and the

Marina to see the dolphins, pods of which followed boats into the Marina.

It was illegal to feed these friendly creatures, although visitors continued to pat, and feed them. With a group of tourists from Japan, Gabrielle watched as the dolphins gathered at the sound of their voices, circling, and swimming close to the edge of the jetty.

It was thought that the dolphins followed the boats in from the ocean to the marina. and when the fishermen went out at the weekend, they threw bait and fish to the pods of dolphins.

Although it was cold, Gabrielle waited for low tide, then walked out to the water's edge, stopping to collect shells of different marine molluscs, all very different in shape and colour. She saw a group of people flying drones over the area, smiling at the children running after the circling drones.

She had packed lunch, and stopped to eat, then, refreshed, she made her way to the Elvis Presley museum. 'Elvis,' Peter, was an enthusiastic Elvis fan, devoting his life to his collection of Elvis memorabilia.

Every room in the suburban house was crammed with Elvis collectibles. Gabrielle was amazed to know that, among the vast collection, Peter had some ninety-seven Elvis clocks, and, she laughed at this, even an Elvis toilet seat.

Leaving the house after a smiling goodbye from Peter, she made her way back to town. She found the local pharmacy and bought several items, then visited the 'Dollar' shop for a camera.

She had booked ahead, and made her way to the Eyre hotel, parking the car and checking in at reception.

Gabrielle had planned to spend at least five days driving from Covell, before her next Agency job at Alice Springs in the beautiful Northern Territory. She would make a leisurely trip of some one thousand, five hundred and three kilometres, via the Stuart Highway, a journey of some seventeen, give or take, hours.

She planned to stop at a motel on the way, probably Port Augusta. She was a seasoned traveler, knowing that every couple of hours she should stop to stretch her limbs.

She had her camera in the car, and would be on the lookout for kangaroos, camels, emus, and wandering cattle. Hitting a large animal could be catastrophic.

Aware too of the road trains, many as long as fifty-five metres. Overtaking one of these huge forms of transport needed a lot of room.

She would stay in Coober Pedy overnight after the five thirty-seven-kilometre drive from Port Augusta, and then on to Alice Springs the following day.

Early the next morning, having filled the petrol tank and two containers with petrol, and stocked up on fruit and sandwiches, Gabrielle bade farewell to Covell. The journey from Covell to Port Augusta was uneventful, taking two hours.

Again, the first stop was to refuel the car and find a restaurant for a welcome cup of coffee.

Gabrielle was aware that the restaurant was mostly filled with Aborigines, who eyed her with curiosity. The next pit stop would be at Coober Pedy, the opal mining town, although the underground dwellings, dugouts, were also an attraction.

The dugouts remained cool despite the scorching daylight heat. The town was well known for its guided trips into the underground mines, and Gabrielle looked forward to experiencing all the town had to offer.

The town was originally called Kupa Piti, an Aboriginal term for, 'White Fellas Hole.'

Gabrielle had booked in advance at the motel, and made easy time to the town arriving at sunset. Much to her surprise, the motel had been built inside a mountain. Gabrielle checked in and was shown where she would spend the night.

The suite of rooms included a kitchen, not that she planned on cooking.

She slept soundly that night, and was up early the next morning having breakfast, so that she could wander around the town before departing on the next leg of her journey.

With luck, she would arrive in Alice Springs around two pm. The car was ready and serviced, and with several opals and small keepsakes from the town, she set forth refreshed. The drive to Alice Springs was hot and tiring, the car leaving a cloud of red dust in its wake.

Although she saw camels and emus on the plains, she was fortunate enough not to encounter any on the road, and she gave a sigh of relief when the town of Alice Springs appeared in the distance.

At the entrance to the hospital, she parked the car.

Chapter Sixteen

Walking up the entrance steps, she became aware of brown stains looking very much like dried blood, liberally spread around. She gave her name at reception and within minutes was being escorted to her room, which was unlocked by using a card key.

Her suitcases were brought to the room by a porter, and making sure she had the card key. Gabrielle made her way to admin. A short wait before she was shown into the Director of Nursing's office, greeted, asked a few questions, and welcomed.

A white clad R/n was summoned, and with a smile, from the D.O.N, she was sent on her way to be shown around the hospital, accompanied by the R/n. This was a large hospital, and the patients predominantly Aboriginal, the nursing staff white Australians.

After the tour, they made their way to the surgical ward, where Gabrielle had been rostered on duty the previous day. A thirty-bedded ward, four patients to each room, and four single rooms for patients needing more intensive care, or considered unsafe to be in the general population, because of a potentially communicable disease.

Certainly, tuberculosis was active among Aboriginal people.

Since Gabrielle had a fevers certificate, she was a valuable addition to the nursing staff. The hospital had a maternity ward, and a psychiatric unit, and Gabrielle knew she would be asked to work wherever she was most useful.

Registered nurses with her qualifications were rare, and she was appreciated because of her versatility. Finally the two made their way to the canteen, where they selected food from the selection on offer.

Gabrielle was surprised at how good the food was, having had years of experience with unappetising hospital food. As they talked, Gabrielle looked around the area, commenting occasionally to her companion.

She hoped that the R/n, Marian Black, would prove to be a friend during the next six months.

Marian was rostered to the surgical ward, so they would cross paths. Again, she slept well, and dressed in Agency uniform, made her way to breakfast and joined Marian, who was also on an early shift.   At 7am, Marian greeted the night staff, introducing Gabrielle.

The ward was well staffed, three student nurses., three enrolled nurses, and the two R/n's. Gabrielle took notes during the handover, then, as the other staff left the office, smiled, when Marian took the drug cupboard keys.

" Medication first, you can have a word with the patients as we go round."

 In the first room Gabrielle said good morning, stopping at each bed to talk to the patient.

Medication round over, they returned to the office, Marian asking if Gabrielle had any preferences, regarding meal breaks or off duty hours. She shook her head.

"I'm here to work, whatever's best forward management."

 "That's a relief, most Agency staff aren't quite as accommodating."

"It's a vocation for me, perhaps not all of us feel like that,"

Time enough to talk about staff expectations. Gabrielle was kept busy with five patients. Mr.' Short Fred', who was recovering from a total gastrectomy.

Looking at the board listing patients' names, diagnoses, room number, and treating specialist, Gabrielle was aware of how easy it would be to make mistakes, given the possibility of confusing an Aboriginal name.

Mr. 'Short Fred' was an example.

Aboriginal lore was a mystery to Gabrielle, and she was aware that unless she spent years nursing Aboriginal patients, they would remain a mystery, given they were a stone age culture.

So different from all that she knew, she would be diligent in her care of her patients, double checking everything she did. Most of the female patients were addressed by their first name since they had no surname. She knew that the word, Ab... origine, was Latin for, 'since the origin', meaning, they inhabited this land first.

Australia's first people. Enough surmising. She had written a worklist and would attend to Mr. Fred first. He was in a single room and sleeping.

She checked and recorded his vital signs, slowed the flow of the intravenous, which currently was delivering a Dextrose saline fluid, and gently checked the abdominal dressing. Mr. Fred remained asleep, which Gabrielle was grateful for.

The operation, to remove his cancerous stomach was brutal and his prognosis poor. He was a known alcoholic, as were many of his tribe's people. In fact alcohol, although banned, was still readily available, and caused much illness, and chaos, among Aboriginals.

She administered an antibiotic via the I.v and noted the time for his next analgesia.

She had brought the liquid nutrition formula Fred's doctor had ordered, a blend of proteins, fats, vitamins, and minerals and polysaccharides, all the micronutrients the body needed, and delivered via a gastrostomy tube, a tube directly into the jejunum.

She scrubbed her hands, having first removed the abdominal dressing, and slowly administered the liquid, using a 50 ml syringe.

Fred slept throughout the procedure. Finally, she redressed the wound, and noted the fluid intake on the fluid balance chart, then, after signing for all procedures, she left the room.

Her second patient, Daisy, was a young married woman who had been attacked by her much older husband. The unfortunate woman had suffered a crippling wound, having had her Achilles tendon severed in the assault.

Gabrielle tended the dressing gently, speaking quietly, although Daisy kept her face turned away and uttered not a word.

Daisy Two, as she was called, in the next bed, had also been assaulted. The cuts on her face were infected, and again Gabrielle attended to the wound, speaking quietly to the young woman.

The third patient, in a single room, was a mid-thirties American man who had been involved in a vehicle accident several days previously.

He had been operated on to remove his ruptured spleen.

Gabrielle attended his dressing, after introducing herself, and assisted him out of bed, into an armchair. He was a smoker, so a physiotherapist worked with him, ensuring deep breathing exercises prevented an onset of post operative pneumonia.

Smokers were always at risk. Pain from their abdominal wound caused them to take shallow breaths, not fully expanding the lungs, and, on occasion, opportunistic bacteria caused pneumonia.

After putting his water jug and glass within easy reach, Gabrielle left him to his own devices, although at his insistence, promised to look in on him before she went off duty.

Mark said he loved her accent, and since his next adventure was to work in London, he wanted to 'pick her brain.'

Laughing, she left the room.

Marian was ready for morning tea, and talking about their morning so far, the two entered the canteen.

Gabrielle listened, as Marian talked about her patients, knowing she might well be attending to them, when next on duty.

Marian had been born in Alice Springs, so nursing Aboriginals, and knowing their culture, was second nature to her.

Gladly, she shared knowledge, talking about the illnesses, and trauma that brought patients to the hospital.

She said the previous day, two warring tribes had fought, using primitive weapons, and more than twenty men and women had been admitted for care. Gabrielle shook her head.

"That explains the blood on the steps when I arrived yesterday."

"Yes, they fight with sticks, anything that comes to hand. Some of the injuries are frightful. Trying to educate the youngsters, and stop the use of alcohol is an ongoing battle".

Making their way back to the ward, Marian added.

"Would you like to catch up, when we go off duty?"

Gabrielle nodded. "Great, what do you have in mind?"

" We can wander around the town, see some of the sights?"

"I'd love that, I'm fascinated with everything I've seen so far."

Tending to her last patient was also a challenge. This teenager had been admitted for ongoing self-harm.

He had slit his wrists and been found before he bled out. He would be transferred to the psychiatric ward when his wounds were healed. Suicide was, unfortunately, a frequent occurrence among the Aborigines.

Soon enough, the shift was over, and Gabrielle handed over the report on her patients.

True to her word, she visited Mark, who was now back in bed, and she spent a short time talking with him.

Marian looked in, and Mark thanked Gabrielle as she left.

They parted ways in the Nurses home, changed into civvies, and met at the hospital entrance. It was a pleasant thirty-five-degree day, and talking, they made their way into the town centre.

Gabrielle was astounded to see, a few streets before the centre, Aboriginals, male and female, lying in the small enclosure obviously fast asleep, surrounded by empty bottles.

Marian explained that this was a common sight.

Aboriginals spent the night drinking, then the day asleep, wherever they happened to fall.

Gabrielle was appalled, to say the least. She was aware that her understanding of the Aboriginal culture was nonexistent.

Furthermore, on reaching the town centre, she realized that the white people thronging the area were cosmopolitan.

American, Japanese, German, and probably Scandinavian, since she was unable to identify the few words she heard.

Gabrielle needed a torch, so they found a hardware store and browsed.

She bought a hot water bottle, at Marian's comment that the nights and early mornings were very cold. Alice Springs was proving to be nothing like what she had imagined.

Marian, still talking, entered a small café where she was greeted by the owner.

Seated, Paul, the owner joined them, inquiring about Marian's health, had she recovered from the cold she'd had when he last saw her?

It was very apparent that Paul cared for Marian and she for him.

He brought three mugs, a plate of carefully chosen cakes and a jug of coffee, which they consumed whilst they talked.

Paul was from Adelaide, so he was interested to hear about her impression of the city. Several groups of people had entered the café, and Paul, with a lingering look at Marian, and a smile for Gabrielle, joined the staff to serve his customers.

Saying their goodbyes, the two young women walked to the Tourist centre, taking brochures of the surrounding attractions.

Gabrielle hoped she and her new friend would have some off duty periods at the same time, so they could visit tourist spots together.

The days passed quickly, no two alike. Gabrielle, who previously believed she was well versed in all things nursing, realised, regarding the care of Indigenous people, she knew very little. Humbling, indeed.

One morning, she entered Daisy two's room, to see the I.v tube lying on the bed, and Daisy, nowhere to be seen. Daisy had gone walkabout. This, evidently, was a frequent occurrence.

Mr. Fred made slow progress, Mark had been discharged, promising to keep in touch, the self-harm lad was transferred to the psychiatric unit, and Gabrielle greeted each day cheerfully.

In the office the second week, she answered the phone, to learn a new admission was on the way.

He had suffered haematemesis, a bleed from the stomach.

This was unusual, being a medical, not surgical ailment. The only available bed was in a four-bedded room. Quickly, she prepared for admission, surprised when the surgical Registrar joined her.

"Morning, Sister, you heard about the admission? He'll go to theatre as soon as he's stabilized, he's been cross matched for blood, will you get a porter to fetch the supply from the Lab?"

"Good morning, yes, of course, anything else I should know?"

He's in a bad way from all accounts, let me know when he gets here."

Gabrielle nodded, and left the room to find Marian. Gabrielle knew little about Henoch Schonlein Purpura, H. S. P. except that it was a rare inflammatory disease of the small blood vessels.

The onset was sudden, with the sufferer experiencing headaches, an elevated temperature, loss of appetite, abdominal pain, cramping, and joint pain.

The unfortunate sufferer could also have kidney, gastrointestinal, and even more rare, central nervous system, brain involvement.

Little was known about H.S.P, although it was thought to be an immune disorder, possibly related to an allergic reaction to certain foods or drugs. Thankfully, Marian had nursed the young man previously and was confident that he would soon be on the road to health.

Gabrielle read the latest entries in the voluminous notes, which had been sent from medical records, surprised to see that he had his sixteenth birthday a week previously.

On admission it was immediately apparent that the boy was acutely ill.

Pale, and sweaty, he groaned and tossed, seeking to relieve his pain. The Registrar, summoned by Marian, arrived and swiftly examined his patient. Morphine had been given via the I.v which the G.P. had performed prior to the boy's admission, needing to cut down into the vein, since his veins were inaccessible because of his collapsed condition.

Gabrielle, with a student nurse, moved a patient from a single room so that the boy could be nursed in isolation. As Dr Lloyd turned to leave the office, the boy vomited, a gush of blood erupting from his mouth and nose. All three were covered, and the nurses quickly turned the stricken patient on his side to prevent him from aspirating vomitus into his lungs,

Dr Lloyd phoned theatre, to prepare for an emergency exploratory laparotomy.

The boy, unconscious, but still vomiting blood, was supported on either side by the two R/n's.

Marian had pushed the emergency bell in the room, and two students appeared, faces paling, as they took in the blood-soaked area surrounding the bed, and both sisters.

"Will one of you fetch linen and a bowl of warm water to wash him. Get his notes, and a permission form for operation, and make sure there's blood for him in the fridge.

Also, see if his parents can be contacted. He's going to theatre, oh, get a gown and a wrist band, too."

Both students were back within minutes, and the boy was prepared for theatre, the theatre porters waiting with a gurney. It was agreed Gabrielle would accompany him, and with her uniform covered by a gown, the three hastened to the lifts.

Chapter Seventeen

Once inside the lift, Gabrielle, feeling for the boy's radial pulse, willed the lift to reach the theatre floor. Swiftly, the gurney was pushed into the anaesthetic room, where Gabrielle left the patient to a theatre R/n and went to don a theatre gown.

All was ready, and the patient was transferred onto the operating table. The Consultant surgeon, and his Registrar stood, gowned, masked, and gloved, whilst the anaesthetist struggled to stabilize the boy.

As Gabrielle moved towards the operating table, the anaesthetist said curtly.

"He's arrested".

Despite defibrillation, epinephrine, and lidocaine being used, no heartbeat could be established and after thirty minutes he was pronounced dead.

All staff, medical and nursing, stood quietly, only the sound of the various machine loud in the quiet space. After several minutes, Mr. Talbot nodded to his Registrar, and they left theatre. Gabrielle was numb.

She checked the time, on the large clock, estimating it had been less than an hour since the boy's admission. Quietly, theatre staff began preparations to clean, having called porters to take the body to the mortuary.

In the anaesthetic room, Gabrielle gathered the instruments sent with each patient to theatre, and with a brief goodbye to the R/ns left the suite.

Despite years of nursing, she was in a state of disbelief. No relatives had accompanied the boy to the hospital, nor inquired about him since his admission.

Slowly she walked back to the ward. Marian was in the office, talking on the phone, eyebrows raised in question. Gabrielle shook her head. Marian replaced the receiver in the cradle and asked.

"Coffee?"

"I could use one."

In the kitchen, they sat, whilst Gabrielle recounted the last minutes of Milo's life.

"Have his relatives been contacted?"

"He was in care, no relatives known."

Both women sat quietly contemplating the life of a sixteen-year-old boy who had no one to mourn his brief time on earth.

The rest of the shift was uneventful, and Gabrielle was glad when the handover was given, and she and Marian left the ward.

They both had the following day off duty, and Gabrielle had been invited to go with Marian and Paul for a drive into Desert Park.

With a group of people of all nationalities, the three took a trail and multilingual audio guide,

choosing to walk the trails rather than use the electric scooters at reception, and made for the sanctuary.

In the gloom were lizards, spiders, and snakes, all easily visible.

The thirteen-hundred-hectare environmental and education facility wildlife park was a tourist attraction.

A living culture, where Indigenous, and non-Indigenous guides showed tourists the spectacular nocturnal sanctuary, with its rare and endangered species.

The trio were captivated by the quolls and echidnas, the rock wallabies, numbats, and little pygmy possums. Once outside, they resumed the trail.

Overhead, they saw free flying birds of prey, owls, curlew, tawny frogmouths, red capped robins, and eagles, many of

whom could be hand fed by visitors.

So the weeks passed quickly with every day new challenges. Although she was glad to have had the experience of nursing in the Red Centre she would be happy to return to Adelaide.

In the solitude of her room that evening, Gabrielle prepared for her final day in the hospital. She had made friends and enjoyed nursing those of a vastly different culture.

Away from the confusion of her feelings for Connor, and her sadness at Olivia's misfortune, she knew her decision to nurse as an Agency member had given her time to collect her thoughts and make wiser decisions.

Her final day was hectic with new admissions, and little time for regret at leaving newly made friends.

That afternoon, she again repacked her suitcases, thankful that having already made the journey once she would have no problem on the trip home. She retired to bed early that night so that she could make an early start before the heat became overwhelming.

The car had a reliable air conditioner; however it used a lot of fuel, and she wanted no part of breaking down out in the middle of nowhere. By five thirty the next morning she was up and showered.

She had brought provisions for the journey and filled both petrol containers with petrol, aiming to drive from Alice to Adelaide with as few stops as possible.

Now that she was ready to go she wanted to be in Adelaide by the following day, stopping for the night at Coober Pedy where she had spent the night on her way to Alice Springs, although it was a grueling drive.

With her suitcases in the car and all checks made for the journey, she left the town, once again heading for the Stuart Highway.

At this early hour there were few cars or big rigs on the road, and at ten o'clock she pulled into a pit stop, unpacked her sandwiches, and enjoyed a cup of coffee from the flask.

On the road again, with a Chopin Etude playing softly, she thought of May's excitement the previous evening when she had phoned with the news that she was homeward bound.

She wondered if Connor had decided that his only option given her long absence, was to move on with his life. It was almost a year since she had seen him. Perhaps absence did make the heart fonder.

With a wry smile, she thought, 'of someone else', laughing quietly, although she was despondent at the thought.

She had no doubt about her feelings, whether the same could be said of Connor she had no idea. At two o'clock, she stopped briefly to get out of the car and stretch her legs.

Transport thundered past now, all makes of cars and big rigs headed in both directions.

She wondered at the lives of long haul drivers, thinking what a lonely and hard life it must be away from family and loved ones.

She at least had nursing companions with whom to share the months away from all that was familiar to her. Life was strange, she mused.

She recalled a member of the English band, the Beatles, saying, 'life is what happens when you're making other plans.'

Thinking, perhaps it was John Lennon.

One of Gabrielle's favourite pastimes when making long car trips, was to imagine Henry the Eighth in the passenger seat, spellbound, as she explained how an airplane stayed aloft in the sky.

Traffic lights, modern buildings, supermarkets, all the everyday things she took for granted.

She imagined telling him of the various medical procedures to combat his weight and heal the ulcers on his legs, as well as the sexually transmitted disease he was thought to have contracted. She smiled, thinking that those who knew her would be puzzled by the way she entertained herself, alone, and driving.

She wondered what other drivers thought about.

No doubt family, their children, a mortgage, the problems at work, the disagreement with a neighbour. She had purchased some American cassettes on different physical ailments and methods of nursing patients with challenging illnesses.

They helped pass the time, and she realised American nursing practice was very different, as was Australian.

She would never forget her first week of nursing at Caringbah, in Sydney.

The drive to work, going down in the lift to confront a Consultant who told his private patient about the following day's operation but failed to tell her, the person responsible for the patient's preoperative preparation. The way Australians shortened words, 'brekkie' for breakfast, 'hozzie' for hospital, 'Sis' instead of Sister, and four bedded rooms instead of a ward with some twenty-five to thirty beds in the same area.

Yes, she had learned a lot during her stay in Australia.

Most of all, she had learned about herself, her own emotional needs, her tolerance for those with challenging personalities with. No doubt she had grown in many ways.

It was hours ago that she had crossed the South Australian border, and familiar landmarks began to appear. Thankfully she had reached Coober Pedy, weary, and looking forward to a hot meal and a long night's sleep.

She was heartened at her greeting by the hotel staff who remembered the lovely young woman after her stopover some months previously.

Her ensuite room awaited, dinner would be served in the restaurant, or if she preferred, in her room. She chose to book a single table and made her way to her room accompanied by a porter with her suitcases.

A hot shower and fresh clothes revived her, and she made her way to the restaurant looking forward to the hotel's excellent food.

She had ordered breakfast for a six-thirty a.m. start in the morning, and after dinner made her way to a park where wildfowl flocked in their journey to who knew where.

She wondered if Connor enjoyed the great outdoors, she knew so little about what gave him pleasure.

Indeed, she wondered if her constant musing on Connor and his life in the many months of her absence was adding to her unhappiness.

He may well have settled his differences with Olivia. It wouldn't be long before she knew. Her routine established; she retired early that night, setting her alarm for five forty-five a.m. and by six fifty she was on the road to Adelaide.

She would stop briefly at Port Augusta and be in Adelaide by the afternoon. She needed to concentrate on the way from Port Augusta. On the outward trip she had driven from Covell, to Alice Springs. Going homeward she would leave Port Augusta and make for Port Pirie, then on to Adelaide.

The scenery had changed from the red and arid plains of the Northern Territory to the lush green pastureland of South Australia. No longer camels and emus, but fields of sheep and cattle. The many small towns she passed through were picturesque.

Occasionally she would stop to photograph something which caught her eye knowing her photos would be reminders of her wanderings. As she drove, she wondered whether May felt as happy as she felt, to see her home again. Home, funny to think she thought of Adelaide as 'home'.

Yet Connor was there, gladly, she would make anywhere he was, home. She tried to quell the thought, she would be devastated if he viewed her with distrust, so hurt had he been by her flight from him.

Better to concentrate on her next job. She would apply to a nursing Agency in Adelaide. She was qualified to work in a general, psychiatric, or midwifery facility, preferably in a large hospital.

By three p.m. she had reached the outskirts of Adelaide, glad to be back in the city she was beginning to know.

At last, she was in the leafy suburb, where May lived. As she parked the car in the driveway the door opened, and May, a smile on her face, met her saying as the two hugged,

"I'm so glad you're home and safe, come in, I've been awake for ages wondering how far you'd travelled and when you'd be here, I've missed you so."

Gabrielle's head was still alive with traffic noises from the eight-hour drive, and with a sigh of relief, she sank into an armchair whilst May brought in a tray, saying,

"Have a cup of tea, then if you're hungry I'll get something substantial to eat, you said you wouldn't stop for lunch."

Gabrielle's s eyes were closed.

"A cup of tea would be welcome, I ate a sandwich while I was driving so I'm not hungry, May."

"Have your tea, then if you want a shower go on up, your bedroom's ready, you'll find towels and the toiletries you left here. I'll bring your cases in."

The shower was refreshing, and Gabrielle, dressed in a tracksuit, rejoined May in the warm sitting room. May was eager to hear of Gabrielle's adventures since last she been in Adelaide, and the afternoon passed with news being exchanged.

 May had heard seen Olivia at the local shopping centre accompanied by a well-dressed man.

'She is stunning, yet, from what you say, she doesn't sound like a very likeable person".

Gabrielle shrugged.

 "The main thing is she's out of my life, what she does now doesn't concern me, although I can't help wondering what's happening between her and Connor. She's no doubt sweetness and light with him".

"After the trouble with Richard, I hoped you and Connor would make a go of it."

"May, Olivia was never going to let that happen, much as I didn't want to go, there was no other option."

Rested, and eager to begin the day, Gabrielle was up before May, preparing to leave before May came downstairs. A note would suffice, and a phone call later.

Closing the front door quietly, she made for the car, listening to the radio as she made the trip into town. She entered the office of the first Agency, smiling at the receptionist, who asked if she had an appointment. Gabrielle explained that she had come to leave her details.

"Miss Stevens next interview isn't till 10 o'clock, I'll ask her if you can see her now?"

At Gabrielle's nod and smile, she knocked on the office door, and within seconds Gabrielle was seated in front of Miss Stevens whilst her C.V was being examined.

"The Agency always has a place for someone as well qualified as you, Miss Graham. There's a dire shortage of R/n's currently, let alone those with your abilities."

"Thank you, I'm keen to start as soon as possible."

The interview was over, Gabrielle stopped at a petrol station then made her way home. The aroma of roasting chicken was enticing, and she greeted May, who said.

"Right at lunch time, I thought perhaps we could have our main meal now and something light for tea if that's okay? How did the interview go?"

"No problem, I didn't need to look for a second Agency, I start tomorrow."

"That soon? I thought you'd take a few days to take it easy."

Gabrielle laughed.

"Onward, and upward, May…"

She had been given the details of her first job, and dressed in a white blouse and navy skirt, standard Agency uniform, she was bright and early next morning before the day staff came on duty.

Hospital staff were well used to temporary staff from various Agencies, she was greeted by the night nurse and told where the off-duty roster was.

She was glad to see that her request for early duties had been accepted.

She wanted to get to know the patients before she would be asked to take over as senior R/n on duty in this mixed ward for neurological and neurosurgical patients.

Twelve patients on each side of the corridor A] neurological patients, and B] neurosurgical patients.

She was rostered to side A, the neurological side of the ward. She had three student nurses working on the shift with her and as the report was read she took notes.

Handover over, she asked the students to begin assisting patients who needed minimal help with showering, she would see to any medications given before meals, then join them.

The morning was trouble free, each student capable of caring for their patients, giving Gabrielle time to read patient notes.

In the four-bedded room, two patients who had suffered severe head injuries in car accidents.

One patient who suffered from Parkinson's disease, and the fourth, a man in his sixties, who had been hit in the head by a cricket ball.

Each man needed care with hygiene, feeding, and toileting.

In the second room, four female patients, two elderly women who had suffered a C.V.A. cerebrovascular 'accident', [stroke.]

One young woman whose skull was fractured in a riding accident, and the fourth young woman an unfortunate sufferer of encephalitis. The two elderly patients were making good progress thanks to early intervention, and would soon be transferred to a nursing home.

The young woman with the fractured skull, was also improving, all three receiving daily physiotherapy, needing less care each day, all intent on becoming independent, although they were full of gratitude for the nurses care.

The patient suffering from encephalitis had just been diagnosed after her initial collapse two weeks previously.

She had been at home playing with her four-year-old daughter, when she fell, causing the child to scream. Catherine's mother-in-law was in the kitchen, and fortunately for Catherine, was a retired R/n. She immediately started C.P.R, and within minutes Catherine had started breathing unassisted, although she remained deeply unconscious, breathing stertorously.

Within minutes, the ambulance had taken Catherine into A and E where she was immediately assessed, I.v infusion commenced, and a neurologist called for consultation. Catherine had regained consciousness, and although pale, insisted she felt well enough to go home.

Chris, her husband, arrived at the hospital, concerned but assured that she felt better although she recalled nothing about the last few hours.

Chapter Eighteen

A few days passed uneventfully, and that weekend his mother took the little girl so that Catherine and Chris could have a few hours alone.

On Sunday morning, whilst having breakfast, Catherine suffered another seizure, and again was taken to A and E. This time Chris insisted that she be admitted as an inpatient, and she complied.

Catherine had begun an intensive array of tests, C.T scans, urinalysis, and blood tests, and the following week was diagnosed as having epilepsy, and with anticonvulsant medication and an outpatient appointment for the following day left the hospital.

Unlike the previous weeks, Catherine was sluggish and uncoordinated. Chris thought that the medication was affecting her speech and asked his mother if anticonvulsant medication would affect Catherine like that.

That evening Catherine suffered a third seizure, and again was admitted to the neurological ward. It was very apparent that epilepsy was secondary to whatever else was going on in

Catherine's head, The neurologists intensified their efforts to see what was causing this young woman's illness.

She was drowsy most of the time, becoming irritable when nurses attended to her, and during all the procedures which thus far had failed to show the cause of her symptoms.

She was scheduled for an M.R.I, the following day.

M.R.I, an abbreviation for magnetic resonance imaging, was a radiology procedure which forms pictures of the anatomical and physiological processes of the body. For many this was frightening, particularly for those with a fear of being enclosed, claustrophobia.

Catherine, however, slept throughout the test only waking as she was lifted into bed. Over several days she became progressively more confused and weaker, exhibiting a marked loss of sensation.

Chris was at her bedside day and night praying for a miracle.

The neurology Consultant had assured him that Catherine hadn't suffered a stroke. Four days after admission with her condition steadily deteriorating, a visiting American neurologist was asked to consult, which he gladly did.

The tests continued, a lumbar puncture, to send cerebrospinal fluid to the laboratory, an E.E.G. (electroencephalography,) to measure the spontaneous electrical activity of the brain.

After a lengthy examination of all available tests and a few minutes asking Catherine questions, he said quietly.

"We'll leave this young lady to rest; we can talk in the office."

Gabrielle, the Consultant, and neuro Registrar entered the office, and the American said simply.

"She has encephalitis, whether it's viral, bacterial, or immunological, will take a while longer to discover."

Encephalitis. An infection of the brain. Gabrielle had hesitantly mentioned this to the Registrar, who disagreed.

She had nursed several patients in Alice Springs with encephalitis and had first-hand experience. The young Registrar's knowledge came from books.

She did not look at him, although as they continued talking, she was aware of his eyes on her.

She was not one to rub salt into a wound. How to treat Catherine was much more important.

Again, the American neurologist was knowledgeable. A bacterial infection should respond to antibiotics. A viral infection, antiviral medication. Rubbing his chin, he continued.

"If it's her own immune system, she's in for a bumpy ride, we're not so familiar with immune causal encephalitis."

Neither was Gabrielle, both patients in Alice Springs had been successfully treated with antibiotics.

Fortunately, the latest batch of results from the Path Lab showed that the infection was due to the shingles virus, Herpes Zoster.

Gabrielle had mentioned to the Registrar, that Catherine had suffered shingles a few months prior to the onset of the first seizure.

He had not replied. Gabrielle was grateful that her flight to the Northern territory had given her the knowledge to nurse Catherine back to health.

The American and Australian neurologists left the ward whilst the Registrar wrote an antiviral regime.

Gabrielle waited, and finished writing. The Registrar commented.

'I owe you an apology, you were right."

"I nursed several Aboriginal patients in Alice Springs with encephalitis, so I recognized the symptoms, and she'd had shingles."

"It was still good call; I'll pay attention to you Brits in the future."

Laughing, he left the office. Leaving her staff nurse in charge, Gabrielle took the medication chart to the pharmacy. She wanted no delay in commencing the medication.

With anticonvulsants, sedatives and corticosteroids, Catherine made a gradual recovery, and several weeks after admission she was discharged with outpatient follow-up.

Gabrielle knew that it would take many months until Catherine returned to some semblance of her former vibrant self.

On the next roster change, Gabrielle had two days off duty and then was allocated to the neurosurgical side of the ward.

She went shopping in the morning, intent on buying a dictionary on neurology. Finding nothing that interested her in Masons, the bookshop, she left the shop to see if the department store over the road offered a larger selection.

She looked across the road, her face losing colour as her eyes alighted on the familiar form of Connor Quinlan, smiling down at the lovely young woman by his side.

Gabrielle gasped, involuntarily, and walked back into the bookshop, eyes blinded by tears. So, both she and Olivia were forgotten. Connor had moved on, to pastures new.

She returned to the car; all thoughts of neurology cast aside. Her hands trembled as she put the ignition key in the lock, and bumpily, she exited the car park, wanting the security of home, of May.

Within minutes she had driven to May's house, where she parked the car in the driveway, waiting until she regained her composure.

The house was quiet. Gabrielle called. "May?"

"Out here, you're back early, did you get what you wanted?"

May entered the kitchen, knowing from Gabrielle's expression, that all was not well with her.

Quietly she set out mugs and put the jug on to boil.

"Tea, or would you prefer coffee? "

"Coffee, thanks." "

"Biscuits, or do you prefer cake?"

"I'm not hungry, thank you, May".

"Are you going to tell me what's troubling you?"

"Why not, it's about time I got on with my life and stop obsessing about Connor."

"You've spoken to him.?"

"No, I saw him when I was leaving Mason's."

May pushed the milk towards Gabrielle, waiting.

"He was occupied, so I left them to it."

"Them?"

"He, and whoever it was he was with. They were so absorbed with each other; he wasn't looking at anything but her."

"You don't know her?"

"No, she must work at the same hospital that he does."

"Gabrielle, it's been months since he heard from you, and you did tell him that you didn't see a future with him while Olivia was in the picture."

"I didn't think he'd move on so quickly, more fool me ."

May frowned.

"Perhaps it's as well, you know where you stand, now, although, I must say I'm surprised; I thought from what you said that he was in love with you."

Gabrielle spent the following day at the library, finding several books on neurosurgical procedures, and looking forward to returning to work.

The neurosurgical patients were diverse and challenging. There were four single rooms on this side of the ward, and two four bedded rooms.

Monday was admission day, and Gabrielle and the three student nurses were kept busy with the admissions, and for Gabrielle, a ward round. During a quiet moment she read each patient's notes.

In room one, there was a young man with a cerebral tumour, for operation the following day. In room two was a fifty-six-year-old man with Parkinson's disease, admitted for surgery the following day.

In the first four bedded room, a patient with epilepsy, another with a brain aneurysm, and two younger men, one with O.C.D, and the other with Essential tremor.

In room four, a young woman with acoustic neuroma, another suffering cluster headaches, and two patients with benign brain tumours.

Gabrielle was surprised to learn that obsessive compulsive disorder, could be treated by so called deep brain stimulation, in which a small incision is made into the skull, and an electrode implanted into the specific area.

Parkinson's disease, and epilepsy were also treated with D.B.S. The day passed swiftly as Gabrielle prepared each patient for upcoming surgery. She had always enjoyed nursing patients with neurological and neurosurgical diseases. They were challenging, and it was rewarding, when the patient left the unit, cured or improved.

It was, indeed, a miracle to see a patient who was unable to drink liquid from a feeder, feed themselves with a steady hand.

Something taken for granted by those not suffering from Parkinson's or Essential tremor.

Gabrielle rejoiced in her ability to be part of a team which brought about such a life-changing circumstance.

After twelve weeks in the neurosurgical ward, Gabrielle was asked to relocate to the psychiatric unit.

She would once again be back in the environment she loved and knew so intimately. As usual, she was given two days off duty before changeover.

On the last day of her neuro surgical placement, she was in the office selecting medication charts for the four hourly medication, when the Registrar appeared.

She smiled, said 'good morning', and continued with her task, concentrating on her work. After several minutes, she suddenly became aware that the Registrar remained, unspeaking, watching her intently.

"I beg your pardon, are you waiting for a particular medication chart?"

"Actually, I'm waiting for you."

"You want to examine a patient?"

He laughed. "I want to talk to you."

Flustered, Gabrielle said. "Something wrong?"

"Do you Brits ever think about anything but work? I want to ask you if you'll have dinner with me?"

He was undeniably attractive. She would go so far as to say, judging by the confusion some of the female staff exhibited whenever he was around, gorgeous. However, she was still recovering from the disappointment of her short relationship with Connor.

Surprised, she replied, 'Dinner?"

"You do eat dinner?"

"Of course, I'm just surprised that… I mean, that you…."

 "Gabrielle, you must have known I was attracted to you, everyone else seems to know it."

'I had no idea, I thought you were just very diligent in the care of your patients."

He laughed at this.

"That's one of the reasons I find you so attractive, you're unaware of your effect on the opposite sex. "

"I concentrate on my work when I'm on the ward. I don't look at the opposite sex as anything but medical staff."

"Noted. So, must I wait until you're off duty?'

"I think I would like to have dinner with you."

"Since we haven't been formally introduced, my name is David, I'm single, and very interested in furthering a harmonious relationship with our English friends across the pond."

Involuntarily she laughed, soon joined by David.

"I really enjoy the Australian sense of humour".

Indeed, Gabrielle had always found a man with a quirky sense of humour appealing. David handed her a card with his phone number.

"May I have your address, then I can meet you this evening".

After he left, Gabrielle walked into the first four bedded ward, all well, likewise the other patients.

There were no problems with intravenous giving sets, all the preoperative procedures had been carried out, so that on the following day, all would go smoothly. She was off duty at three p.m. and made her way home.

May, ever cognizant of Gabrielle's mood, smiled.

"A good day at work?

"May, you would never believe…..one of the doctors at work asked me to have dinner with him."

May laughed. "Gabrielle why so surprised, you're a beautiful young woman."

"Yes, but… I don't know, I wasn't looking for anything."
"Sweetie, it'll do you a world of good, the saying…'all work, no play,' is very true. You've been so wrapped up in work lately."

"I know seeing Connor with another woman was a shock, still it gave you the push you needed to forget him."

"May, what would I do without you?"

"Probably drink less coffee. So, what's the young man's name, and when is he calling for you?"

"Tonight, seven, and I've nothing suitable to wear."

"Give me a few minutes, then we'll go and find something beautiful."

There was no shortage of department stores to shop in, and having tried on several, Gabrielle chose a pale blue muslin dress with a scoop neckline. Shoes and a small evening bag completed the ensemble.

 Gabrielle laughed when May remarked.

"Retail therapy, such a lovely way to spend a few hours."

"I'll have a shower, then I'm ready put on some light makeup, and get dressed."

May smiled. "You've plenty of time, nervous?"

"I'm not, he has a lovely sense of humour. I'm really looking forward to spending time with an attractive, intelligent man."

May was quietly happy for her young friend. On the stroke of seven, May answered the door to a tall handsome young man.

"Do come in; Gabrielle's upstairs, I'll let her know you're here."

Upstairs, she knocked on Gabrielle's door.

"He's here, he's gorgeous, and he's waiting."

Gabrielle laughed. "May, you're incorrigible."

"Have a lovely evening, you deserve it."

"Thank you, I will. "

It was soon apparent that David was an attentive companion. They talked, laughed, and compared the differences in the English and Australian medical systems.

 Too soon it was almost midnight, and David drove to May's house. Parking the car just short of the house, he turned to her.

"That was an amazing first date, you're a keeper."

Gabrielle laughed. "David, it's a good job I don't take those remarks seriously."

Although he laughed, she sensed he meant what he said. She thanked him for a lovely evening, and as he leaned forward to kiss her, averted her face so that his lips met her cheek.

"Woe is me, nevertheless, I'm not dissuaded."

"Good night David, and again, thank you."

May met her at the door, smiling at Gabrielle's glowing eyes and softly flushed cheeks.

" You enjoyed the evening?"

"May, he's such a sweetheart, so ready to please. I'm rather concerned that he wants more than I can give."

"Already? What makes you say that?"

"The way he looks at me, some of the things he says."

"Such as?"

"He said he's been wanting to ask me out since the first time he saw me in the ward. May, that was weeks ago."

"So.?

"He didn't think I'd accept; he waited all those weeks..."

"I didn't take much notice of him, although I saw several of the student nurses looking at him with the kind of expression I can only describe as 'love struck."

Laughing, Gabrielle hugged May. "Two days off, luxury, we must plan something good for tomorrow. See you in the morning, and May…."

Smiling, May responded, "Gabrielle."

"Thank you."

"For…"

"For being such a good friend when I needed one."

"Off to bed with you, sleep well."

Sleepily, Gabrielle prepared for bed, thinking about the evening, and wondering if David would be content with friendship.

Somehow she didn't think so. Rather than sleeping in the following morning, Gabrielle was up and ready for the day at seven a.m.

Over breakfast, May confessed that it was years since she been to the Adelaide Art Gallery, and that should be their first port of call.

Adelaide C.B.D was twenty minutes away, and they soon parked the car, and walked into the gallery.

The Victorian building was established in eighteen eighty-one, and housed paintings, sculpture, photographs, metalwork, ceramics, jewelry, furniture, and textiles.

Gabrielle was especially interested in the Indigenous and Torres Strait Islander art.

Wandering through the rooms, admiring exhibits and reading about the work being displayed took several hours, and Gabrielle remarked that there was still so much more to see.

Chapter Nineteen

They decided to drive to the Adelaide Hills for lunch, stopping in the German village of Hahndorf, which was established by German Lutheran migrants escaping religious persecution in Prussia in eighteen thirty-eight, and named Hahndorf after their ship's Captain.

The picturesque village was the oldest surviving German settlement in South Australia. Gabrielle had been told that there were still direct descendants of the thirty-eight founding families.

Gabrielle shopped for souvenirs, and then they made their way to the Hahndorf Inn.

They stopped several times on the way, admiring the German Village shop, the giant nutcracker statues, and the toy train moving along the red tracks lining the ceiling. The shop boasted the largest cuckoo clock in Australia.

They bought fudge in the Fudge shop, and smiled at the concrete sheep and sheepdog on the pavement in the main street.

Finally arriving at the Inn, they were seated, and after studying the menu, opted for the 'Taste Of Germany' platter, which, when it arrived, proved large enough for three or four diners.

The atmosphere was electric, Hahndorf was a popular tourist destination, and always crowded. Gabrielle had visited the beautiful Adelaide Hills on several occasions, however because she was short of time, had not visited Hahndorf.

The restaurant was full, and as they ate, they looked at the wait staff in Tyrolean costumes.

Finally, with much of the platter remaining, the two called it quits, and returned to the car. Gabrielle had never seen anything similar to Hahndorf and thoroughly enjoyed the trip.

The phone was ringing, stopping as they entered the hall, and on playing the messages,

Gabrielle heard David's voice, asking if she would go to a concert he had tickets for at the Entertainment Centre.

Smiling at May, Gabrielle returned his call, and it was agreed they would meet at the venue. After the concert David walked with her back to her car and waited while she found the keys.

"Gabrielle, my parents are here from Melbourne, I told them about you, and they'd love to meet you".

Gabrielle wondered what meeting his parents meant for him, it seemed he wanted to make their friendship into something more than it currently was. Perhaps she was being presumptuous?

"David, forgive me if I'm misreading this, what does my meeting your parents mean to you?

"Gabrielle, from the first time I saw you on the ward, I was attracted to you, since getting to know you better, I realise that you are…"

"David, before you say anything else, I should tell you I'm not looking for a permanent relationship. Friendship, certainly."

He smiled. "I value your friendship. We don't know what the future holds, still, I can dream, can't I?"

" I enjoyed the concert, let me think about meeting your parents."

She drove home, wondering if her love for Connor would ever be resolved.

May was in bed when Gabrielle quietly entered the hall and made her way upstairs. Before she fell asleep, she wondered what May would think about David's suggestion.

The following morning she was tired, having slept poorly. Her dreams were of circles, yet, not complete circles, spheres, incomplete. May greeted her in the dining room.

"Late night?"

"No, I kept being woken, dreaming about the strangest things."

"Something troubling you?"

Sensible May, always knowing when Gabrielle was concerned about a situation.

"May, I've only been out with David on two occasions, yet last night he asked me to meet his parents."

"You don't want to?"

"May, it can only mean one thing, he's serious about our being together."

"Gabrielle, is that so bad, he's a lovely young man, why not meet his parents?

He's in a profession which gives people back their lives, he obviously cares for you, he's attractive, intelligent, and well educated.

Most young women would be delighted if a man like that showed the slightest interest in them."

"He's not Connor."

"Oh Gabrielle, Connor's made his choice, you can't spend the rest of your life grieving for what might have been. "

"May, I love him, I long for him, nothing makes sense without him."

May said nothing, indeed, there was nothing to say.

May was aware as never before of the depth of Gabrielle's love for Connor, understanding that meeting David's parents meant letting Connor go.

A man like David would not invite a young woman to meet his parents unless he was intent on a committed relationship. Quietly, the two sat contemplating what had been shared, until Gabrielle began clearing the breakfast dishes.

"May, we have all day before I'm back on duty, let's go to the zoo?"

"Why not, I haven't been to the zoo for years."

The drive to the zoo and parking the car was soon accomplished, and they opted for an interactive experience, going to the enclosure to see the lions first. The pride was so much more majestic than either woman had imagined.

They gazed enthralled, at the Sumatran tigers; the lofty giraffe, and the Orang Utans.

They were looking forward to seeing the Giant Pandas. After a quick lunch they visited the snake house.

 The giant green anaconda, a non-venomous boa constrictor which killed its prey by, as its name implied, constricting the unfortunate victim and cutting off its oxygen supply, was magnificent.

The Pandas, oblivious of their many admirers, were sitting close to each other, eating the specially grown bamboo.

 Gabrielle read that Pandas lack digestive enzymes, which allow other herbivores a wider selection of plants, thus, bamboo shoots, stems, leaves, and roots, were the only plants Pandas tolerated.

Gabrielle was enchanted by the giant tortoise, telling May that she had owned a tortoise, named Fred, whose name was painted on his shell. Fred, unfortunately, was given to wandering.

May laughed when Gabrielle continued.

"One day, Fred was nowhere to be found, I looked everywhere. The following morning I found Fred in the front garden, with a note attached to his shell, saying, 'please keep Fred at home, he's eaten all our lettuces.'"

They both laughed at that as they made their way to the enchanting Meercats.

Deciding that five hours of animal watching was sufficient for one day, they returned to the car to make their way homeward.

A quiet evening was spent at home, and Gabrielle made the evening meal which they ate sitting in front of television watching 'Panorama'.

When they said goodnight they hugged, and Gabrielle said.

"I'll be gone by six thirty, so I'll see you when I'm off duty tomorrow."

"What time will you be home?"

"Depends what's happening, it's a different placement, the psych: unit, so I've no idea".

She slept well that night, looking forward to working on the psychiatric unit. She had realized years ago that she loved the challenge of nursing patients with complex psychological issues.

She was up bright and early the following morning and at the hospital by six thirty a.m. It was a beautiful day and she greeted other staff as she made her way to the psychiatric unit.

She was assigned to P. Two, and as she walked along the corridor, she could hear a female voice, raised in anger.

Entering the office, she was greeted by night staff. She introduced herself, taking her seat at the desk ready for handover.

Staff nurse West gave the report, then the students left the office, and West gave Gabrielle a more detailed report on each of the twelve patients.

Gabrielle knew that this unit housed those suffering from anorexia nervosa, and held group therapy for outpatients with severe phobic disorders.

Little was known about anorexia or bulimia, although they were classed as mental disorders, and in recent years it became known that there was a genetic susceptibility.

Sufferers of anorexia developed patterns of eating, restricting their intake of some foods, and avoiding others which were' fattening.

' Certain characteristics were observed in those with an eating disorder, they were perfectionists, obsessive, compulsive, often neurotic, with low self-esteem issues, and seen as emotionally' absent'. .

Socio cultural influences also contributed to the illness. Unrealistic expectations for impressionable youngsters with body image concerns.

'You can never be too thin.'

Your skin must be blemish free'.

The media all stressing that to be successful in life, one must look as near perfect as possible. Gabrielle was aware that more than one million Australians suffered from eating disorders.

She had nursed patients with both conditions prior to leaving England, and was familiar with the therapeutic methods used in supporting patients. West said she was on duty for the next four nights and would see Gabrielle the following day.

The staff nurse on duty, named Johnson, had worked on the ward for several years, so Gabrielle took some time to read patient notes before she met them.

On the ward she introduced herself to the young women, and the two men, noting that several had nasogastric tubes and that they were fed using a fortified supplement. She knew several patients were off the ward, in the library and occupational therapy.

She had agreed to work split shifts so that she could work with patients at different times of the day, enabling her to interact with them and observe their behaviour in response to various stimuli.

At lunch time, staff monitored patents who were known to be skillful at hiding food. No bags of any kind were allowed in the dining room, and each patient knew that staff would check their pockets, and even their shoes on occasion to ensure that food had not been secreted there.

The regime was familiar to her, with little difference from other eating disorder facilities she had worked at.

Severely ill patients were not allowed to shower unattended,' water load', or exercise.

Food and fluid charts were meticulously kept.

She wanted to talk to patients before she held the first group session.

The oldest patient was a twenty-three-year-old woman who had been hospitalized on numerous occasions, and was one of four, who were tube fed.

The youngest, also female was fourteen, with a history of anorexia from the age of seven; both males were teenagers. The day passed quickly, and when writing the report, Gabrielle was content that she knew what she needed to know in order to interact with these unfortunate people.

The following day she was on duty early, anticipating an interesting day ahead. Staff nurse West reported that it had been a relatively quiet night, all patients conforming to expectations, with the exception of William Marshall.

He had been on day leave, returning to the ward in the early hours of the morning, uncontrite and smelling of marijuana. Gabrielle read his notes as West gathered her belongings and left the ward.

After breakfast, Gabrielle asked the group to meet in the room set aside for therapy, which they did. She had her diary and various leaflets which she thought the patients would find educational.

William knew better than to remain in bed, although he was surly and contributed nothing to the conversation.

Gabrielle began as was usual in group therapy, and since she was new to the patients, gave her name and a brief account of who she was and what she did.

Then each patient gave their name and the length of their stay in the unit.

The twenty-three-year-old woman, Eve was eager to talk about her new acquisition, a guitar. Since Gabrielle had no musical experience, the subject was somewhat confusing.

She knew that several of the young patients were professional sportswomen, and asked if anyone wanted to tell the group about their experience of their illness and the impact on their life.

Eve, for whom hospital was a second home, was first to volunteer.

"I had a happy childhood, my elder brother and my parents doted on me, I was an 'A' student at school, and my life was great."

"I was chosen to represent the junior school when I was twelve, I won every event I was in, except for the high jump".

" No matter how much I practiced, and I couldn't have tried harder, I failed again and again. My coach said I needed to drop some weight; I was too heavy."

"So I did. I cut out different food, I went for three hour runs every day. I kept a diary so I could keep an eye on what I ate. I weighed myself, before I ate and afterwards."

" I started wearing clothes that were loose, so my parents didn't know I was losing weight. If I gained an ounce over forty-eight kilos, I panicked."

" My hair began to fall out, I had arrhythmia, because there was no potassium in what I did eat, according to my doctor.

   Gradually, all that mattered was losing weight. I got so weak, I couldn't run, but I still exercised"

"My family took me to different psychiatrists, and I spent more time as an inpatient than I did at home. "

"I'm frightened of gaining weight, although until I'm at my goal weight of forty-eight kilos, I'll be hospitalised."

Given that she was one hundred and seventy centimetres, she was still painfully thin, gaunt, even.

  Gabrielle asked if antidepressants had made a difference.

"Yes and no, I don't think of killing myself as much as I did before, only when I'm really fed up with my life, but I'm sick of getting headaches, feeling giddy, having an upset gut."

Chapter Twenty

Several in the group agreed. Alison, another patient being tube fed, added,

" I know that dieting or binging is a way of dealing with emotional turmoil, every psychiatrist I've ever seen, has told me that, but while I can't always control what happens to me, I can control what I eat or don't eat."

This time, everyone agreed, and Gabrielle said.

"So, we must understand how to manage negative emotions and life's traumas without causing life threatening illnesses."

"Using food to reward, or punish oneself, is for many, a lifelong battle. Food not only fills our stomachs; it fills an emotional need in us. "

"We eat to comfort ourselves, to reward ourselves, and, with anorexia, and bulimia, we do not eat, perhaps, to punish ourselves.

" Since so little is known about eating disorders, treating both illnesses is difficult. As well, celebrating with food is accepted in so many cultures."

"Birthday party food, wedding celebration food, all are very much part of our culture. I'm sure we've all heard of parents who are concerned about their toddler not wanting to eat, until eventually it becomes a struggle."

" Even a toddler can control his or her parents by their willingness to eat what's on the plate, or refuse, and watch how their behaviour affects these otherwise powerful adults."

"I worked on a paediatric unit, where there were at least four or five so called, 'failure to thrive 'infants. An eighteen-month-old boy was admitted one day, severely underweight, and if you can imagine it, depressed ."

 Eve said, "depressed?"

"Yes. He wouldn't eat, wouldn't play, he cried most of the day and when he was awake at night, so yes, he was depressed. "

Alison asked. "How was he treated?"

" He was tube fed, I read his notes as soon as I had the opportunity, and it transpired that he was the fourth child of an eighteen-year-old mentally challenged single mother, who left the toddler outside the pub in his pushchair, and gave him a bag of potato chips when he cried."

" The social worker was told that he was also given beer or whatever his mother had been bought."

He would eat potato chips, but refused everything else."

Gabrielle was aware that the group were visibly affected by the story.

She continued, " I'm telling you this, so that you understand. The use of food to control one's own emotions, or as this little boy clearly demonstrated, other people's emotions, is a complex and powerful….for want of another word.. tool, a weapon, a strategy..."

Matthew asked, "what happened to the kid?"

"He spent a year on the ward. Different foods were introduced gradually into his diet, and the dietician devised a menu especially for him, even cutting vegetables into animal shapes to tempt him.

He was given ice cream, which he loved, different fruit, and strawberry jelly which he ate, and sometimes played with."

" Every staff member, nurses, allied staff, made eating fun. Gradually, the naso-enteric tube was removed, and he started interacting with the other children.

The staff loved him. He was cuddled and made a fuss of, and gradually he began to understand that he was an important part of everyone's life. "

Alice smiled. "Then what, don't say his mother took him home?"

"No, one of the nurses on the ward adopted him. Incidentally, so were his two sisters and his brother. "

"By different families?"

William, this time.

Gabrielle smiled. "Welcome to the group, William."

Everyone, including William, laughed. "Okay, I was well out of order…that's what pot does to me."

" To answer your question, William, yes, the children were adopted by different , loving families, and it was agreed the children would grow up knowing each other."

"I stay in touch with Diane, Archer's adoptive mother, if you like, I can read her letter, and show you a picture of Archer."

She fetched her bag from the nurses station and returned to the group, passing the photo of Archer to William.

"That was taken when Archer was admitted to the ward."

 Passing him the second photo.

" That was on his second birthday."

"Diane sent this on his first day at primary school."

The group, impatient, crowded around William, exclaiming.

 Eve said, " he doesn't look like the same child, his bones are sticking out, in the first photo."

" He's so beautiful in his school photo, it doesn't look like the same child."

Gabrielle nodded.

"That's the nature of anorexia. Archer was taught how to eat; it wasn't a choice."

The group sat silently, each feeling the force of the words, left unsaid.

Gabrielle knew that telling Archer's story had made a significant impact on everyone. They were happy that Archer had finally been accepted into a loving family; yet sad, that their own lives were so out of control.

Gabrielle asked if anyone wanted to talk about whatever they wanted to share. the group were silent.

William said, " it really makes you think, doesn't it, that a baby can get depressed."

Gabrielle's voice was soft. "It's been recognized for decades that babies deprived of affection become depressed, they express their emotions by crying, initially, then not accepting food or fluid, they fail to gain weight…"

William said, "Please, enough, that's hard to hear."

"Yes, even harder to nurse, but, William, take another look at Archer's primary school photo."

"I'm happy he found someone who loved him."

"As were we, and now, we'll leave it 'til tomorrow. Just a reminder, I'm here, if anyone wants to talk. "

The group thanked her, and she returned to the office, to write notes. She turned around, at the knock on the door, to see William standing there.

"Sister, you said if anyone wanted to talk to you.."

"Certainly, I'll be with you in a minute. "

" I wanted to apologize for being a prize twat."

Gabrielle laughed. "That's hitting the nail on the head."

"I'll apologize to the night staff too. I know what I'm like when I'm stoned."

"The thing is, you know the effect it has on you, and you can choose not to let it change who you are. I know you said all your friends smoke dope, and what they're like when they smoke, you don't need to give in to peer pressure."

William nodded. " My old man said he'd kick me out next time I came home stoned. Brave, seeing I'm twice the size he is."

He smiled. " I know that what you said, about controlling people by choosing not to eat is true. I've done that as long as I can remember, until it's gotten to the point that I get sick when I eat, and I'm frightened."

"William, think about this, you realise you need help, and you want to eat. That's powerful, you've taken the first step."

" I'll get the dietician here, and together , we'll think of a menu you'll enjoy… small steps.." Smiling, William thanked her, and left the room.

Gabrielle knew that the tough guy persona William adopted, hid the true person within.

She was off duty when the patients had their evening meal, however, the nursing staff were well equipped to care for those with eating disorders.

She spent a quiet evening with May, knowing David was meeting his parents, disappointed that she would not be with him, although he respected her decision, aware that his feelings for her were nor reciprocated.

He understood that her relationship with Connor still weighed heavily on her mind, and he had decided that he cared enough for her, to accept whatever relationship she was prepared to enter into with him.

The following day, Gabrielle met with the dietitian, and both treating psychiatrists at the staff meeting. She had prepared her notes, and the meeting was informative.

 Each patient was discussed, treatment and medication reviewed, and ongoing options for each patient, in response to their weight gain or loss.

None of the patients being tube fed had gained sufficient weight, therefore, the regime would continue. Gabrielle knew they expected this, yet they still fought staff 's efforts to help them overcome their fear of eating.

Anorexia had such a hold on their thinking, even those being tube fed, wanted to know what was in the formula, and , if not constantly observed, would try to find a quiet location, where they could purge, or exercise, squats, jumping jacks, anything to shed a few ounces.

  The fear of weight gain was toxic for every patient on the ward. Gabrielle never ceased to be surprised at the game playing, the aggression , the tricks that anorexic, and bulimic patients used, to resist gaining an ounce.

In the mornings staff meeting, Eve's psychiatrist had talked about Eve being moved to a secure unit, she was losing weight rapidly, despite the specially prepared formula, and extra smoothies. The only explanation was that Eve was, somehow, managing to dispose of the smoothies.

The group met in the therapy room, the flowing afternoon. Linda, a seventeen-year-old had been admitted that morning.

As usual, each group member, including Gabrielle, introduced themselves, and gave a brief account of their journey through the traumatic world of eating disorders.

Linda was encouraged to talk about herself, and a familiar story was told.

Linda had become fascinated with ballet, as a four-year-old.

By the sixth grade, she was fully accustomed to weigh ins at ballet school, to fainting, because she was hungry, to not eating sugary or starchy foods, and loading up on protein, fruit, and vegetables.

She confessed that students were praised for losing weight, and made to weigh themselves daily, to ensure their weight remained stable.

By the age of ten, she was making herself vomit, after eating, and using laxatives, and she was exercising for three or more hours a day.

She told of her teacher criticizing her, because she had gained several ounces, and that she was made an example of. She admitted that she had suffered several bouts of gastroenteritis.

Matthew asked her if dancing was worth the pain she endured, on a daily basis. She was quiet, and the group waited, silently.

With tears in her eyes, she replied.

"No, because I was too tall to become a professional ballet dancer. I felt so guilty, knowing my parents each took on several jobs, to pay for classes, ballet shoes, tights , leotards, and whatever else I needed. I hated myself, I was a selfish, self-absorbed, brat."

As she spoke, she was removing her trainers, and socks. Holding her legs out in front of her, and her feet aloft. The group stared, appalled.

On her left foot, the big toe was out of joint, positioned over the second toe, and every toe was disfigured.

On her right foot, there was a bunion on her big toe, and, like the toes on her left foot, each toe was disfigured. There were scars from previous injuries, and abrasions.

She smiled, bending to put her shoes , and socks back on.

"The physical pain was nothing, compared with the emotional and psychological pain, Dancers get used to physical pain., and eventually, psychological pain".

"However, that didn't register, I set my sights on being a dancer, and if it killed me, so what?"

Eve asked if all ballet dancers had problems with their feet.

"Not just their feet, I've got a bad back, tendonitis, and my ankles have been sprained so many times, I've lost count."

Quietly, the group sat, contemplating the life of athletic athletes, which Linda certainly was.

Gabrielle said quietly. "Thank you, Linda, for your honesty, everyone here knows how difficult it is to accept the damage anorexia is responsible for in your lives."

"You're all aware that you'll remain in the unit until you reach the weight most beneficial for you, we've talked about the reason for not having scales or mirrors in the unit."

" About the necessity for cognitive behavioural therapy."

Matthew sang out, "You are what you think."

Smiling, Gabrielle continued.

"The value of meditation, aromatherapy, and all the other supportive therapies. How you move forward in this process is up to you".

" Staff can support patients to a certain extent, the hard work and acceptance that each one of you has an eating disorder is your responsibility."

The rest of the shift passed without incident, and leaving the unit that evening, she felt that progress was being made.

She had one more week in the eating disorders unit, before she was allocated to another ward. She had two days off duty, and planned to spend them with May, exploring the Botanic Gardens and the Cleland Wildlife Park.

They took turns to take photos, holding a koala, and feeding the tame kangaroos. The following day, Gabrielle drove to the city centre alone, intent on kayaking along the Torrens.

May had things she wanted to attend to. The scenery along the river was breathtaking, and she felt the stresses of the last few days slip away.

Returning the kayak, she found a bench under a huge eucalypt, and sat down, still exhilarated from the row.

Watching pedestrians walking along the banks of the Torrens made her aware that she was one of the few people on their own.

Couples with strollers, teenagers in groups of three or more, not one single individual. She wondered what Connor was doing with his new love, and if he ever gave her a fleeting thought.

Whether Olivia felt the pain she felt at the loss of Connor, or had she too made a new start?

The laughter of a child brought her back to the present and looking at her watch, she saw she needed to get moving. The sun was setting as she drove back to the suburbs and in good time parked the car and entered the hall.

May greeted her, calling her into the kitchen from which came the aroma of apples, baking.

May asked, " Did you have a good day?"

"Yes, anything I can help with while I tell you what I got up to?"

"No, dinner's ready, and there's an apple pie in the oven. We can eat in the lounge if you like?"

May had made a cottage pie and cauliflower cheese, and, trays ready, they moved into the lounge room.

While they ate, they talked and watched the news. Gabrielle cleared the plates, after the first course refusing dessert, and putting the kettle on to make tea.

Gabrielle entered the ward the following morning with mixed feelings, knowing it was the last week on the unit.

The office was crowded. The Registrar, Consultant psychiatrist, Staff nurse West and a student nurse all standing around the desk..

They greeted her quietly, and as she moved to the desk, Dr Palmer, the Consultant said.

" Sister, I'm sorry to be the bearer of bad news. Eve was found in the bathroom this morning, having hung herself in a cubicle."

Gabrielle gave an involuntary intake of breath.

"I told her yesterday she was being transferred today, and she said she wouldn't go, she would discharge herself."

"My only option was to section her, and get staff to keep an eye on her."

No one spoke. The twenty-three-year-old had preferred suicide to being treated in a secure psychiatric facility.

It weighed heavily on all present, and the effect on the remaining patients was traumatic. That day, all the staff sat quietly with patients who expressed their feelings in different ways.

Most cried, and talked of their own feelings about their illness. Gabrielle asked the group if they wanted to meet in the therapy room and silently they assembled.

No one spoke, and after a few moments, Gabrielle said.

" If anyone wants to talk about anything at all, please do."

The group remained silent.

"We're all shocked by Eve's suicide; at a time like this we can only offer comfort to each other".

"Eve struggled with her illness for years, despite ongoing care and support, it was her decision that she no longer wished her life to continue along the same path".

"For myself, I'm desperately sorry that we couldn't help her. The staff are beyond sad."

" We will let you all know about the funeral arrangements, and rest assured, staff are ready to offer all the support we can to you. "

They continued to sit quietly, then Matthew said.

" I thought she'd jump at the chance to get intensive therapy, it's a crappy thing to do."

Several in the group were outraged, while others agreed. Gabrielle waited until it was quiet, then said.

"Suicide by its very nature is confronting and makes those left behind sad, angry, bewildered, all the emotions you're feeling now. How could that person do such a thing.?"'

"Life is precious, yet people worldwide take their own lives every day. When it happens in the context of an illness like anorexia, it's confusing because the person has all the support possible."

All I can say is that for many, anorexia changes the sufferer's brain patterns. They are no longer able to make rational decisions because it's all too overwhelming."

" Eve had been anorexic since the age of twelve, eleven years of hospitalization, medication, psychotherapy, every treatment available, yet, she was so firmly in the grip of the disorder, she could no longer see a way through.

She's at peace now, and that's what we would want for her."

"More so now, staff are only too ready to talk, or just sit with you if you wish."

Chapter Twenty One

The following days passed with no further untoward events, and on Friday evening, Gabrielle said goodbye to the patients and staff, promising to let them know where she was next assigned to. Her thoughts as she drove homeward were troubled.

Losing a patient to suicide was traumatic for everyone who knew the person, Gabrielle always ruminated on what more she could have done. May was visiting a friend, so Gabrielle had the meal that May had left for her, eating the salad, and with most of the food left untasted, covered the plate with plastic wrap and put it back in the fridge.

Her appetite always deserted her when she was troubled. There was a message from May, saying the Agency had phoned, would she return the call. She phoned and listened to the snatch of classical music before she heard Rebecca's voice.

" Gabrielle, good to hear from you, how are you?"

"Well, thanks, and you?"

"Busy, as always. I phoned, first, to see how you are, and secondly, to ask if you would consider working in Victoria?"

"Victoria?"

" I know it's a long way from home, however , this small hospital needs an R/n who's multi skilled, and yours was the first name I thought of."

Gabrielle was silent for a minute, then replied. "Let me sleep on it, Rebecca, I'll let you know tomorrow."

Victoria, she knew Melbourne was the capital city, and that it was a multicultural destination for people all over the world. She went to bed early that evening, she would see May in the morning.

She was awake at seven the next morning, and when she heard May stirring, she prepared a tray of tea, and knocked on the door. May was sitting up in bed, and greeted her with a smile.

"I didn't wake you last night?"

"No, I was tired, so I went to bed early."
"What have you planned for today?"

"Rebecca asked me if I'd consider working in Victoria."

" Victoria, what's in Victoria?"

"I'll find out today. May, have you been to Melbourne ?"

"Years ago, such an exciting city, too much for me, 'though, I'm a country girl at heart."

"This is in the country and evidently it's just a small hospital. I'll have a shower, and catch up with Rebecca. It sounds interesting, although leaving Adelaide so soon isn't easy."

May smiled. "If anyone's more than capable of taking on new adventures, it's you."

"Let's hope you're right."

Rebecca had a photo of the hospital waiting for her.

"Matron Jackson is old school; she's been there over twenty years. The hospital is in the small town called Andover, I think there's about a hundred something residents."

|It's a typical small Aussie country town, a local doctor, chemist, a small grocery shop, and there's a country market at the end of the month, from all accounts it's a safe place to live."

Gabrielle asked how many beds the hospital had.

" Matron told me they have two beds for geriatric short stay patients, two paediatric beds, and twelve mixed bed for surgical, medical, and obstetric patients.

Any patients considered in need of more than the hospital can offer, are sent to Nhil or Melbourne. Limited x ray and Path Lab: facilities, of course."

"There are several enrolled nurses, one R/n on nights and Matron, although, from what I can make out, she doesn't do any nursing care. What do you think so far?."

"How long is the job for?"

"Gabrielle, as short or as long as you want, they're desperate for a competent R/n."

"I'll take it then; I didn't want anything that tied me up for months."

"You're a life saver, I thought I'd never find anyone."

Gabrielle had some items she wanted from the chemist and the bakery, then she made her way home.

May had the kettle on as soon as she heard the familiar sound of Gabrielle's car. Carrying a plate of sandwiches, she asked Gabrielle to bring in the tea tray, asking, "how did you go?"

"May, I took it, if I'm not happy, I can leave, there's no contract apart from with the Agency. Evidently, they've been trying to engage a triple certificate R/n for ages."

" You'll never be out of work, I'll certainly miss you, but Andover's not that far, three hundred something kilometres from Adelaide, so we can stay in touch. David will miss you."

"May, I feel so badly about David, I've hardly given him a thought, he'll find someone who wants a relationship with him if I'm gone."

"I couldn't agree more, he won't have any trouble finding someone, he's a lovely young man."

"True, he's just not….."

"Connor."

Both women said simultaneously, and laughed.

"May, you know me so well…"

Gabrielle had several days to contemplate her next job, and she and May made full use of the time.

On Sunday Gabrielle packed the car, bid a fond farewell to her friend, and watched Adelaide disappear in her rear view mirror.

The drive was easy, taking a little over three hours, and at one thirty in the afternoon Gabrielle entered the small town, and followed the sign to the hospital.

There were staff parking spaces, and she left the car and entered the main entrance.

Matron Jackson was summoned by the secretary, and after being greeted, Gabrielle followed Matron Jackson to her comfortable sitting room, where a tray with teacups, a teapot, and cake, was placed on a table.

Matron said, "the tea has just been made, you said you'd be here by one thirty, so I was prepared. "

Seated, Matron said. "I'm so glad you decided to join us, this is a small hospital, however you won't be bored, there's always something happening, typical small town accidents and casualties."

Talking, they finished their tea, and Matron took Gabrielle over to the ensuite room reserved for registered nurses.

They had discussed her off duty, and she learned that she would work opposite Sister Blake, who was married and lived with her family on a farm just out of town.

None of the four enrolled nurses were married, and all lived in town. Gabrielle was on duty the next day, Monday, at seven am. to four thirty pm, then Matron was on call until the night staff came on duty at eight p.m.

Gabrielle unpacked her suitcases, the room was large, and comfortable, with a double bed, and a large armchair, a bar fridge, which was stocked with milk, butter, and a whole meal loaf.

In the small cupboard beside the fridge, there was a cupboard with staples, jam, marmalade, and Vegemite, an item Australians used instead of the Marmite she had known from childhood.

It took a couple of minutes to walk into town from the hospital. At the grocery, she bought fruit, a jar of coffee, teabags, and some muffins.

Most of her meals would be eaten in the staff dining room, with her few purchases, she continued along the high street, looking at the notices of upcoming events. One in particular took her interest.

A rodeo, to be held the following weekend. Gabrielle would request an off duty period, she had always been fascinated by rodeos, not an English pastime. She made her way back to the hospital, her purchases were unpacked, and she put the jug on to boil.

Matron had told her that the water in the large water container was distilled. Making a pot of tea, she returned to the armchair in front of the window, watching the birds splashing in the birdbath. She wondered if there was a mobile library in Andover.

She was thankful for her reliable car, perhaps there would be some sort of tourist attraction, although the drive to Andover had not looked promising.

At six o'clock, she joined several staff on their way to the dining room. The enrolled nurses, at first thinking she was a relative of Matron, smiled, but did not speak to her. Seating herself, she said. "Let me introduce myself, I'm Sister Graham and I'll be working with you."

"Sorry, Sister, we knew an Agency R/n was coming, but we thought it was tomorrow."

" I'm Katherine Fraser and my mate is Jill Scott".

"Neither of us live in the hospital, it's only you, Sister, and Matron, who has a flat in the nurses quarters. We've been hoping that the Agency would come up with some enrolled nurses, it's either really quiet here, or we're snowed under."

As soon as the meal was finished, Gabrielle returned to her room to phone May. There was no reply, so she left a message.

She watched the news on television, wondering how different nursing in Victoria would be. She had applied for her Victorian nursing registration months previously, never expecting to move from South Australia.

Such is life, she thought, and her life since coming to Australia was nothing like she had imagined it would be.

Challenging, exciting, confronting, and with her love for Connor unfulfilled, often melancholy.

She was determined to put any thought of him out of her mind, and not feed her passion by speculating on what he was doing , and with whom he was doing it.

She, who taught others how to change or block unwanted thoughts and feelings by replacing them with positive thoughts from happier times, was guilty of obsessing over something she had no control over. Connor. She recalled a patient in a group therapy session saying to the girl sitting near her.

' You know he's taking up space in your head, and not paying rent?' and everyone laughing.

Gabrielle smiled. How true, Connor was a constant in her thoughts, and there was never resolution. The following morning at breakfast, she remembered Matron saying that Doctor Connell did a round every Monday, and she was on the ward before seven a.m. Sister Ames the night duty R/n greeted her, smiling.

The handover took a short while, then Gabrielle was introduced to each patient in the two bedded and four bedded rooms, Ames giving a history whilst Gabrielle took notes.

Nothing complicated, two geriatric patients waiting for a permanent placement, no children in the room reserved for paediatric patients, and twelve beds for mixed surgical and medical admissions.

The current patients were all mobilizing, several postoperative patients were due for discharge, and the medical patients improved and possibly for discharge that day.

Gabrielle recalled the enrolled nurse commenting that the hospital was quiet, or staff were 'snowed under.'

That afternoon, Doctor Connell arrived, Gabrielle was introduced to him, and with Matron , the ward round commenced.

To say Doctor Connell was brusque to patients was an understatement, not that Matron seemed surprised by his manner.

He told one patient, ' it's about time you got back to work', emphasizing the word 'time,' and a second,' 'your wife will have to shape up now you're going home.'

Gabrielle, thinking he was joking, laughed, and then, realising he meant what he said , looked at Matron who avoided eye contact.

She observed Doctor Connell more closely as the round proceeded. He was in his mid-sixties, she guessed, of small stature, with a high pitched voice.

Closer to him, she could smell a mixture of nicotine, and less obvious, alcohol.

Matron, who had worked with Doctor Connell for decades, seemed to notice nothing amiss.

Gabrielle's senses were alerted, although she decided to give Doctor Connell the benefit of the doubt until she had worked with him , and was able to assess his behaviour over a longer period of time.

Chapter Twenty Two

After the round, he told Matron, 'I'm away 'til Tuesday evening, any emergencies will have to go to Nhil.'

No medical cover, not a good situation for the registered nurses on duty, or Matron.

For the first time, Gabrielle felt a sense of doubt and prayed that no emergencies would be brought to the hospital while Doctor Connell was away. The patients for admission came in on Tuesday afternoon..

 Uncomplicated minor surgery and medical conditions which should not be difficult for a competent doctor. On Wednesday morning, phone calls to Doctor Connell's home were unanswered until after lunch, when Doctor Connell appeared.

 The first two patients for minor surgery had been prepared since early Wednesday morning, and were relieved that they would be operated on, and, all going as expected, discharged possibly that evening.

Minor ops theatre had been set up by Gabrielle on Tuesday, and she accompanied the first patient who was scheduled for the excision of a large lipoma on his thigh.

The local anaesthetic was swiftly injected, and Connell proceeded to excise the lipoma, which bled freely.

Connell's surgical skills could be described as adequate, and finally the patient was ready to return to his room, swiftly replaced by the second patient, who had the huge abscess on the back of his neck incised and drained.

Doctor Connell did not speak during either procedure, apart from asking Gabrielle for certain surgical instruments

Having finished the operation, he threw his rubber gloves on the surgical trolley and without a word, left the small theatre.

Gabrielle made certain the patient was ready to go back to his room, assuring him he could ask for an analgesic, if he had pain at the wound site.

She washed the surgical instruments, and put them in the small sterilizer, all the surfaces of the trolleys used were cleaned with an antiseptic fluid; the surgical drapes and gowns were neatly placed in the linen skip, and with a last look around, she closed the door, content that the room was ready for the next minor operation. As she worked, she thought about Doctor Connell.

In all her career, she had never encountered such a graceless individual as Ronald Connell.

He was abrupt with his patients and certain members of the nursing staff, and he seemed disinterested in the work he performed at the hospital.

Matron had said he was married with adult children, he was a proficient golfer, and he had surgery in town.

He often left his wife behind to go on golfing tournaments, leaving the small town without a doctor.

Gabrielle wondered why he continued to stay in Andover, he seemed not to be happy with his work there. Unfortunately the townsfolk relied on him and did not appear unduly put out by his surly manner towards them.

Since most of Connell's patients had been treated by him since childhood, Gabrielle assumed they were accustomed to his manner.

His manner she could live with, his absence was a problem, placing the burden of patient responsibility on the trained nurses.

Gabrielle had never worked in a hospital where there were no medical staff available, furthermore, Matron spent most of her time away from the hospital, leaving decisions concerning patient care to the R/n on duty.

Gabrielle wondered if Rebecca, the Agency owner, knew of the situation at Andover hospital.

Her gut feeling was that Rebecca had no idea. She decided that she would keep a diary of events at the hospital and make photocopies of certain medical notes, where patient or staff safety was potentially compromised.

She had a good idea that this was an illegal practice, however, how else to protect herself, and the patients who put their trust in her?

The following days were uneventful, and Gabrielle settled into the pattern of the hospital, although she remained alert, and watchful.

Matron appeared in the office one morning, with the news that Doctor Connell was taking a month's sabbatical, and that

Doctor Milstead would be available until his return. Gabrielle wondered why doctors in their late fifties, early sixties, were still working as a locum, instead of having a practice of their own.

Milstead seemed a kindly enough man, laughing and joking with his patients. He was staying in the town and unlike Connell, he was readily available.

The round on Monday morning was uneventful, and Doctor Milstead departed, saying he would be at the hospital bright and early the following morning for surgery.

Gabrielle prepared the first woman, a thirty year old married woman for a tubal ligation. She had three young children and did not want a fourth.

Drowsy after the premedication, the patient slept, and Gabrielle and an enrolled nurse pushed the gurney into theatre, where they were greeted by Doctor Milstead.

A spinal anaesthetic was administered, and the patient continued to sleep through the minor procedure. The operation over, and no others scheduled, Doctor Milstead thanked Gabrielle, and left the hospital.

The patient was returned to her bed, and the day continued smoothly. Gabrielle had two days off duty, and early on Wednesday morning, left Andover and drove to Adelaide.

She was glad to catch up with May, and hear her news. The days passed quickly, and on Thursday evening, Gabrielle returned to the hospital, and after a quick shower went to bed.

The following morning, Sister Ames gave handover, and then reported on Mrs. Dean, who had been operated on the previous Tuesday.

"She hasn't passed urine, and Doctor Milstead is in Adelaide until Friday, so he'll review her when he's back. "

"She hasn't passed urine since when?"

 Ames said, "since Tuesday, preop, she's just been catheterized"

Gabrielle , confused, asked, "are you saying she hasn't passed urine since before the operation, despite being catheterised?"

"No, Doctor Milstead said sometimes that happens."

Gabrielle shook her head. "On the contrary, that isn't a postoperative complication."

Ames nodded, but offered no further comment and left the office.

Gabrielle took her notebook, and Mrs. Dean's notes, and went to the room where Mrs. Dean was.

The young woman was sleeping, but woke, when Gabrielle took her wrist and felt for the radial pulse. Gabrielle checked the drainage bag, not surprised to see it was empty.

The woman was feverish, and her pulse was fast. Something had gone badly wrong.

Gabrielle pulled back the bedlinen, and again, was not surprised to see that the woman's abdomen was distended.

Given that she was obviously dehydrated, had a fast pulse, an elevated temperature, had not passed urine since prior to the procedure, and her abdomen was distended, it was very apparent that urine was leaking into the abdominal cavity.

Gabrielle assisted Mrs. Dean to sit up and drink a glass of water, then she commenced a fluid chart. Sister Ames had said Matron was away and would be back that evening.

Back in the office, Gabrielle read the post operative notes, seeing that, according to Doctor Connell, the tubal ligation was accomplished successfully. She found the Deans phone number and dialed it, relieved to hear Mr. Dean 's voice.

Not wanting to alarm him, she asked if he could come to the hospital when he had a moment. He assured her he would be there in the next ten minutes. She met him at the hospital entrance, and took him to the office.

" Your wife has had a postoperative complication, and I would like your permission to have her transferred to Adelaide."

"Adelaide… what happened?"

"We don't have the facilities here to investigate, she can be in the Royal Adelaide by this evening, of course, you can go with her."

"Okay, whatever's necessary, my mother will look after the children."

He left, and Gabrielle phoned the Royal Adelaide, and asked the receptionist to put her through to the gynecological ward. The call was put through, and she spoke to Sister Mortimer, explaining that she would like a patient transferred to the ward.

The circumstances were unusual, and she had taken it upon herself to inform the patient's husband, since the doctor was away and the postoperative patient needed urgent assessment She apologised for this extraordinary departure from the usual protocols, however circumstances dictated it.

Sister Mortimer was surprised, then she assured Gabrielle that she would let the Registrar know at once and she would arrange transport and prepare for Mrs. Deans' transfer to the ward.

In the office, Gabrielle made copies of the notes and put them in her hold all, then welcomed Mr. Dean who had arrived back at the hospital.

He was relieved to know his wife would be sent by ambulance to a major hospital, and was ready to go with her.

Within the hour, the Deans were on their way to Adelaide, and Gabrielle was reassured that whatever had gone wrong would be addressed.

That evening, when she wrote her ward notes, she made certain that everything she had undertaken regarding Mrs. Deans' transfer was written comprehensively, finally making a copy of her written notes. Whatever happened, she had documented evidence of the pre, and post operative notes. Memories were unreliable, documented evidence crystal clear. When Matron returned that evening,

Gabrielle waited for an hour, then sent an E/n to ask Matron to come to the office, and twenty minutes later Matron, in pajamas and dressing gown, arrived in the office.

"Forgive the attire, it's been a long day."

Gabrielle was too professional to comment, and told Matron of what had transpired prior to Mrs. Deans' transfer to the R.A.H, and that in the absence of medical or senior nursing staff, she had taken it upon herself to act.

She added that she had phoned Sister Mortimer a short while ago, and that Mrs. Dean had gone straight to theatre, where a tear in her bladder had been repaired.

She was back in the ward with an intravenous infusion in situ, antibiotics given I.v, and her catheter draining urine satisfactorily.

All going well, she would be returned to Andover after the gynae team had reviewed her the following morning. Matron made no comment, then, at the office door, she said,

"Good, she'll be back tomorrow, I'll see you in the morning

Gabrielle gave the report to Sister Ames, who asked,

"What made you decide to transfer Mrs. Dean?"

"There was no urinary output, she was dehydrated, and febrile, and her abdomen was distended, it wasn't difficult to come to the conclusion that urine was leaking into the abdominal cavity."

"I wouldn't have had the nerve, I knew something was very wrong, but Matron didn't seem too bothered and Doctor was away."

When Gabrielle went to bed that night, her sleep was disturbed, and at five thirty the next morning, she went for a run before breakfast. Exercise always helped her calm her demons.

Mrs. Dean was fortunate that Gabrielle had worked in major hospitals, and was experienced enough to pick up signs of an impending disaster.

If the unfortunate woman had been left until Milstead returned to the hospital, urine leaking into the abdominal cavity would eventually cause peritonitis, potentially life threatening if left untreated. With antibiotic cover, a catheter in situ, intravenous infusion, and the tear in her bladder repaired, Mrs. Dean should make a full recovery.

Doctor Milstead came to the office just after Mrs. Dean had returned and was being put to bed.

He stopped at her bed, smiling, and said.

"So you deserted us for the big city?"

Mrs. Dean , alert and unsmiling, replied tersely, "I don't know what I would have done, if Sister here, hadn't been on duty. "

Unfazed, Milstead said, "We all appreciate the Agency Staff, they're very skilled, because they have a lot of experience in big hospitals, we'll soon have you up, and about."

He made no reference to the bladder tear, although Gabrielle was aware he read Mrs. Deans notes from the R.A.H. very carefully.

Back in Mrs. Dean's room, Gabrielle helped her up, and into the armchair, fetching a footstool.

"Peter and I are in your debt; I dread to think what would have happened if you hadn't been here."

" Perhaps in future go to Adelaide if you or the family need surgery, the facilities are superior."

"Sister, your experience saved me from serious harm, if not something worse."

"Thank you, and as Doctor Milstead says, you shouldn't have any more problems. You're drinking enough fluid to take your antibiotic orally, so I'll take the I. v out and you can move around more freely."

Several days later, Mrs. Dean, accompanied by her husband was discharged, and that day, a bouquet of flowers arrived at the hospital for Gabrielle, with a note which read,

"Our home is always open to you."

Since Gabrielle was the only staff member to receive a gift from the Deans, she took the flowers to her room, she saw no point in advertising that no one else was acknowledged.

She had the following two days, Friday and Saturday off duty, and looked forward to the rodeo on Saturday.

No other staff member was going, so after lunch, she dressed in jeans, a knitted sweater, and boots, and drove to the venue outside town.

There was a large crowd gathering, and having bought a programme, she took a seat in the crowded stand. First on the programme, was bull riding, and, at two o'clock, the Grand Entry, where the stars of the show were introduced to the crowd, got underway.

She knew the bulls were specially bred, and the cowboys and cowgirls were not locals, coming from miles around.

First on the programme was the team roping, and Gabrielle watched as two veterans brought a calf down in a few seconds.

Steer roping followed, again the animal was roped in seconds. Horse racing next, with skilled riders riding their mounts around the ring. Bareback riders on horses, followed, then steer wrestling, with men and women competing, which was a crowd favourite.

Finally the bull riding. Gabrielle watched the chutes as the first cowboy lowered himself down onto the eight hundred kilo bull and placed his hand in the nylon plaited rope

The bull had a Flank strap which caused discomfort and made it buck .

The rider had to remain on the bull's back for eight seconds, not touch the bull with his free hand, and not be bucked off, to avoid disqualification.

Gabrielle marvelled at the skill of the riders and the ferocious way in which these huge, muscled animals twisted and turned, kicking and bucking. The crowd roared and cheered for their favourites, and the afternoon sped by.

Gabrielle thoroughly enjoyed the show. At the hospital, she was in time for dinner, and seated alone, she remembered the cheers from the spectators and the thrills of the bull riding.

She spent the evening looking at the many photocopies of medical notes she had amassed, very aware that in the event of legal action being taken against the hospital or a staff member, she would have medical notes of patients surgery, and medication prescribed, to support her own written notes.

Never in all her years of nursing in England had she thought of such an action. Certainly in the large hospitals in Adelaide and Alice Springs the thought had not occurred.

Country hospitals, however, were a vastly different prospect. She admitted to herself that she was appalled at Mrs. Deans' negligent surgery, and the lack of care postoperatively. she was not a doctor, and it was not within her purview to transfer a patient from one medical practitioners care to another, yet, she had done just that.

With no support from medical or senior nursing staff, she had acted in the best interest of the patient. However, would that be take into account, if the Deans decided to seek recompense for the negligence and she was summoned to court to explain her actions.

Chapter Twenty Three

She did not doubt that they would support her, however was that sufficient, and if not, was it possible that she could be deregistered?

Apart from phoning Rebecca, at the Agency, and confiding in her, Gabrielle was completely isolated. Never had she felt so distant from her workmates, she knew Matron Jackson would not lend a sympathetic ear, if indeed, she understood the depth of Gabrielle's despondency.

Unwilling to abandon the job, she wavered between returning to Adelaide, then, recalling Mrs. Deans' plight, determining to stay and remain vigilant, however hard the toll on her mental health.

Thankfully, she could return to Adelaide on her days off, and the common sense support of May in whom she trusted unconditionally.

The comment made by the enrolled nurse, that the hospital was quiet, or the staff were snowed under, often came to mind.

Thankfully, there were no untoward incidents in the coming weeks, and she settled into a routine, although she remained watchful. Doctor Milstead departed, and Doctor Connell continued as before.

Although regularly unavailable, Gabrielle considered him more competent than Milstead concerning surgical procedures, however the fact that he was absent so often, and completely unavailable in the evening scared Gabrielle.

An elderly man with a history of Chronic Obstructive Airways disease had been admitted at the weekend, and Gabrielle read his voluminous notes, indicating that years of chronic bronchitis and emphysema had finally brought him to his knees with C.O.P.D.

With a sinking heart, she realised that Andover was not equipped to care for him. At the round on Monday, she raised the possibility of transferring him to a facility better equipped to care for him.

"Nonsense," was Doctor Connell's response, "he's at home here, he knows us and we know him."

Matron, as usual, contributed nothing to the conversation, and the round continued, with Gabrielle taking notes. Gabrielle took it upon herself to nurse Mr. Francis, ensuring that the two oxygen cylinders were full, and that his medication, bronchodilator, and steroids were readily available .

The E/n Gabrielle had worked with at the start of the week, told Gabrielle she had a sore throat, and would be absent the following day.

 Matron passed the news on to Gabrielle, saying that the E/n had flu like symptoms, and had sent in the doctor's certificate. Gabrielle worked that day with the enrolled nurse whom she had met in the dining room previously, and who was assigned to the ward.

Mr. Francis, who had felt well enough to shower himself with supervision, the day before, refused his evening meal, and Gabrielle went into his room to ask if he would prefer a bowl of soup, and some toast. To her dismay, he was sneezing and cyanotic, his lips blue.

She took his temperature and pulse, and listened to his chest, thinking he had obviously picked up an infection from the similarly affected enrolled nurse.

His temperature was elevated, and his pulse fast, and since he had a chronic airways disease, it was difficult to pick up any different sounds.

She commenced a two hourly T.P.R chart, and asked the E/n to let her know if Mr. Francis temperature rose any further.

She phoned Matron, whose answer machine was on, and returned to Mr. Francis' bedside, checking his oxygen mask was delivered a steady flow.

He was anxious, and despite the oxygen, he struggled to breathe.

Gabrielle returned to the office, and phoned Connell's residence. Mrs. Connell answered the phone, and Gabrielle asked to speak to Doctor Connell.

"He's unavailable at the moment."

Gabrielle said. "Mrs. Connell , Doctor Connell's patient, Mr. Francis, whom he admitted to the hospital with a chronic lung condition, has an elevated temperature , a fast pulse, and despite having oxygen, is struggling to breathe."

"I'm sorry, my husband isn't able to come to the hospital now."

"Mrs. Connell...

The phone call was disconnected. Gabrielle was at a complete loss on how to proceed, back in Mr. Francis room, it was apparent that he was distressed, adding to his inability to breathe.

The E/n was at his bedside, holding his hand, and both nurses were aware that without medical intervention, Mr. Francis was doomed.

Gabrielle sent the E/n to Matron's flat, and when she returned alone, left her to comfort the dying man, and ran to the office to phone the Connell's residence again.

This time, the call went through to voice mail. There was no locum available, and Gabrielle knew that Mr. Francis would not survive a three hour ambulance trip to Adelaide.

She had asked Doctor Connell to prescribe a sedative which would not depress his respiratory system even further, and thankfully, he had.

Gabrielle took the medication chart, glass phial, and a syringe and swab in a receiver, into Mr. Francis' room, and the E/n checked Mr. Francis's' medication chart, and the phial, then Gabrielle injected the medication into Mr. Francis thigh, and within minutes, his breathing slowed, his eyes closed, and he slept. Nurse Barrett did a quick ward round, reporting that all was quiet.

At eight p.m. Sister Ames came on duty and walked into Mr. Francis room, her face pale, as she took in the situation.

Leaving the enrolled nurse with the sleeping patient, Ames followed Gabrielle into the office and was told of the evening events.

She asked if Doctor Connell or Matron had seen the patient, unsurprised when Gabrielle shook her head.

"Will you be in the nurses quarters tonight?"

Gabrielle nodded.

"Yes, call me if you need some moral support, I'll stay for a while. He had the Midazolam at seven o'clock, and he's as comfortable as it's possible to make him. Neither Matron nor Connell is rousable so you're pretty much on your own."

Ames said. " Mr. Francis has been Doctor Connell's patient for years; he relies on Doctor. Still, I wish Mr. Francis had been transferred to Adelaide as you suggested."

" He lives alone, his wife died several years ago, and they had no children, so he's fond of the Connell's."

Gabrielle forbore to criticize Matron or Connell, and told Ames she would stay with Mr. Francis for a while.

Nurse Barratt went off duty and Gabrielle sat quietly by Mr. Francis bed listening to his laboured breathing and sad for him.

He had told her he was a mill worker, and had smoked a pack of cigarettes a day since the age of twelve.

He had attempted to give up, at his wife's urging, because of his frequent bouts of bronchitis, and in the last few years, emphysema.

When she died, his reliance on nicotine increased, despite his worsening chest problems.

At eleven p.m., she took his hand for a moment, then adjusted the oxygen flow, turned down the overhead light., and left the room.

Sister Ames thanked her, grateful for her support, and Gabrielle walked to the nurses home.

Unsurprisingly, she slept poorly, and was late for breakfast, making her way to the hospital at seven a.m. still eating a piece of toast.

Matron never came to ward until eight thirty, so Sister Ames greeted Gabrielle, and gave the report. All patients had slept well. Mr. Francis had died at two a.m. with both night nurses at his bedside.

Ames said. " He just stopped breathing, one minute you could hear him all over the hospital, and then it was quiet. I'm thankful he had the Midazolam; his last hours were more peaceful than if he had been awake."

She was pale, and had obviously been weeping, as had the enrolled nurse. Mr. Francis had been a favourite in town, and both nurses had known him and his wife, when she was alive.

When the night staff exited the office, Gabrielle left a phone message for the undertaker, and then phoned Connell's residence, leaving a message.

Gabrielle said a quiet farewell to Mr. Francis, aware that the mood on the ward was sombre since the absence of activity in Mr. Francis room; and the sound of his breathing no longer obvious could only mean one thing.

Matron put in a brief appearance when Gabrielle was with the undertaker, and when Mr. Francis ' body had been removed, and Gabrielle returned to the office, she said. "It's a blessing that Mr. Francis is at peace now, and with his wife "

Gabrielle chose not to reply, saying, "There are several admissions later today, if you want to be informed."

"No, Sister, I'm sure you can manage. Nurse Osbourne is back on duty, so we're up to capacity. "

With no further exchange, Matron left the office, leaving Gabrielle to wonder at the complete lack of emotion shown for a man she had known for years.

As always, Gabrielle had photocopies of Mr. Francis latest notes, medication, and made certain to take her bag to her room at morning tea, and put the papers with the rest of the documents, into her locked suitcase.

Doctor Connell did a quick round, and made no mention of Mr. Francis, apart from echoing Matron's sentiments. In the office, he told her he would be away for a few days and Dr.Crawford would be on call.

Once again, a locum, who did not know the patients and would only work in the hospital for the period of time that Dr. Connell was absent.

Gabrielle had Tuesday and Wednesday off duty, and followed the familiar routine of driving to Adelaide when she was off duty on Monday, having worked an early shift.

She and May had agreed, on Gabrielle's previous off duty, to drive to the Barossa Valley, stay at the motel, and book a hot air balloon trip.

On Tuesday, they were up bright and early, preparing to be at the site two hour before sunrise.

They both dressed in warm clothing, and flat shoes, although they knew that the burner in the balloon gave off considerable heat and they wouldn't feel cold.

The balloon was lying on the ground, when they arrived, and they watched as it was gradually inflated; the basket, which was lying on its side, slowly becoming upright..

They took photos of the rainbow coloured balloon before being helped in. It was a strange sensation, floating slowly away from the ground, the mist over the fields and trees dissipating as the sun rose.

Gabrielle knew that hot air balloons fly because hot air rises, being less dense than the cooler air around it, so the balloon floated on the cooler air.

The burner heated the air in the balloon until it became hotter than the air surrounding it. Once that happened, the balloon began to rise, reaching a height of several hundred metres.

The balloon went where the wind took it, and since the wind blew in different directions, at different altitudes, by ascending and descending, the balloon went in the direction the pilot took it.

The view from such an altitude was magnificent, with vineyards, vast areas of green meadowland, and stands of trees. Again, both women took photos and committed the sight to memory.

As they watched, the sun rose, and from above the clouds they could see the Barossa Ranges, and , in the distance, the sea. May, who had a fear of heights, was exhilarated, and laughed, when Gabrielle asked, "still scared? "

May, over a thousand feet in the air, shook her head, laughing.

After an hour, the balloon gently descended, landing smoothly. May hugged Gabrielle.

"If it weren't for you, I'd be at home, working."

" Instead, let's go and see what the motel has on the menu for breakfast".

After breakfast, they drove to the Barossa Valley, famous worldwide for its wine. The scenery was spectacular, and May took photos, as Gabrielle drove to the Barossa Valley Chocolate Factory.

Chapter Twenty Four

The interior of the factory was huge, and there were displays of chocolate, beautifully arranged, as far as the eye could see.

They were fascinated by the twenty four hour chocolate wall, where liquid chocolate ran in a fountain down a specially constructed wall, both day, and night.

They delighted in watching the chocolatiers hand crafting chocolate, through the glass in the artisan kitchen.

Fudge, peanut brittle , honeycomb, all used in the creations, in the massive chocolate production kitchen It was a culinary adventure, and a delight to the senses, for children, and adults.

In the gelateria, they chose from the twenty two flavours, smiling at the excitement of the many children crowded around the display.

The aroma was, May said, 'to die for,' and they made their way around the factory, looking at the huge displays of koalas, skillfully crafted chocolates, and desserts.

Belgian chocolate was used for all the factories products, and at the shop, both May and Gabrielle bought gifts to take with them.

They were told there was a chocolate making workshop which May was keen to try when Gabrielle was off duty in the future, as well as the wine and chocolate pairing at the Vineyard Cellar Door.

Birthday parties were held at the venue, a magical experience, said May, whose grandchildren had celebrated a birthday there and been delighted with the day.

The next destination was the Allerlei, the German name meaning 'all kinds of things,' a shop run by volunteers, where locally grown fresh fruit, vegetables, homemade jams, cakes, slices, and chutneys, were for sale, as well as hand knitted jumpers and retro tea towels.

Before they left the area, they drove to the Cheese Company, admiring artisan made cheeses which were authentic and traditional.

They watched through the viewing window, as the various procedures commenced, starter cultures, coagulation, cutting and stirring, then the cooking, salting, and hooping processes.

Again, both were fascinated to watch artisans at work. Finally, it was time to leave the Barossa, and they talked about the day, as they made their way home, deciding to book a day tour when Gabrielle was next in Adelaide.

Gabrielle worked a late duty on Thursday, and made her way to the ward ready for handover. Sister Owen was on duty, and greeted her asking if she had enjoyed her days off.

This was the second time Gabrielle had met Deidre Owen, and she had liked her on sight. There was an air of fragility about the R/n which Gabrielle found intriguing.

Several discharges and three admissions meant there were no empty beds. Both the elderly ladies had been transferred to an Adelaide aged care village, and Owen said Dr. Crawford was on call.

She had worked with him on previous occasions, and, in response to Gabrielle asking whether he was reliable, replied,

"Yes he is, if you mean does he answer his phone, and will he come if he's needed, however he's somewhat eccentric."

"In what way?"

"It's difficult to describe, he was involved in a car accident several years ago. I didn't know him then".

"Milstead was Dr. Connell's locum whenever Dr. Connell was away, and I never had a problem with him."

"Dr. Crawford, however, is absentminded, he doesn't always write scripts correctly, or he'll get a patient's name wrong, and the R/n's have to remind him of anything he's forgotten, before he leaves the hospital."

"Is he trustworthy?" I don't like to ask, however, if he's unreliable, I'd be happier knowing."

"Just keep your wits about you, when he's here, I'm not sure whether his behaviour is head injury related, or he's just getting older, and forgetful."

"He suffered a head injury?"

Owen nodded. "Yes, he had a thriving practice in Adelaide, then after the accident, he was away for over eighteen months, and he relocated here with his wife and two daughters."

"How long will Dr. Connell be away for?"

Owen laughed. "That's anyone's guess, he says a week then he's gone for three, he'll be retiring soon, he's made a fortune since he's lived here."

"Oh?"

" The doctor here gets paid on how many patients he has, in his G.P practice and at the hospital, the more patients, the bigger the salary."

"Really? I never knew that."

"We live and learn, I'm the town gossip." She laughed.

"I wondered if you'd like to have dinner with me some evening, I've been meaning to ask."

Gabrielle nodded, "I'd like that, I usually have my evening meal in the dining room, and spend the evening in my room, it'll make a nice change, thank you."

"No, thank you. I do the same thing at home, read, or watch television, so having an intelligent dinner partner is great. I do enjoy company, here's the address, around seven, tomorrow?"

Gabrielle smiled, and nodded, taking the slip of paper.

Owen grinned. "Then I'll love you, and leave you."

Gabrielle was taken aback, thinking it an odd comment. So Owen had looked at her off duty, and knew she worked an early shift tomorrow. She wondered if Owen was lonely, or wanted to talk about what went on in the hospital. Tomorrow, she would know.

The early shift went smoothly, and Gabrielle went off duty after handover, and dressed in civvies, for a trip into town. She wasn't sure what she should take Owen, did she drink wine, spirits, or was chocolate a better option? She bought a large box of chocolates and a bunch of flowers, and browsed in the newsagents, looking at various magazines.

A slow walk back to the hospital left plenty of time for getting ready, so she unlocked the suitcase, and looked at her notes, thinking she would be happy to shred them, when her contract at Andover came to an end.

Shortly before seven, she found her way to Owen's cottage. It was a picturesque sight, set alone, and bordered by fields of yellow rapeseed, and in the fields beyond, sheep peacefully grazing.

Deidre was at the door and welcomed her, standing aside to let Gabrielle in. The interior was white shiplap, and the antique brick exterior of the cottage was reflected in the fire place.

Reclaimed pine floors gave an added patina. Gazing round, Gabrielle noticed a spinning wheel in the corner by the window seat.

"I didn't expect this, it's so beautiful."

"It's been in the family for years, my grandfather bought in when he married my grandmother, which was in the early nineteen hundreds. It's been passed down, and I'm the lucky owner now, if you can call that luck."

Gabrielle raised her eyebrows. " You don't like Andover?"

" Andover drives me nuts, but I won't rent the cottage out, and I can't leave it untenanted, so I'm stuck here."

After Gabrielle was shown the rest of the cottage, they went into the beautifully appointed kitchen, and Gabrielle helped take various dishes into the dining room.

Over dinner, Deidre continued to talk about the hospital. Gabrielle listened, but did not comment, although her experiences since she had joined the staff were less than positive.

Deidre asked Gabrielle whether working with the Agency was lucrative, surprised when Gabrielle replied that it hadn't been her main concern when she joined the Agency.

She enjoyed the opportunity to travel around Australia, and working with Aboriginal people and Torres Strait Islanders in Alice Springs had been educational and confronting.

"I'm fortunate that I can go home to Adelaide and May, with whom I live, on my days off."

Deidre frowned, but didn't comment.

After dinner Gabrielle helped clear the dishes, then they returned to the sitting room.

Deidre had an antique gramophone, which had belonged to her grandparents, and asked Gabrielle if she would like to choose a vinyl record from the stack in the glass fronted cupboard

. Looking through the selection, Gabrielle pulled out a popular country song, after which, Deidre chose a romantic record, and to Gabrielle's dismay, turned the lights down, holding her arms out, inviting Gabrielle to dance.

Embarrassed, she said. " I don't dance with women."

"There are no men here."

"Then I'll be a wallflower "

"Your choice, I'll put the kettle on, will you have a cup of coffee?

"Thank you, I must say, the spinning wheel is lovely, was that your grandmother's?"

"Would you believe my grandfather was the spinner, he raised Angoras, and clipped their wool, and after sorting and preparing it, he spun it and sold it to boutique sellers all over Australia."

" Hang on, there's a few skeins in the chest in my bedroom."

Returning, she passed the mohair bundle to Gabrielle, who took it, enchanted by its light fluffy texture. The wool was dyed in a rainbow of different colours.

"He was a master of his craft."

Gabrielle agreed, then as the long case clock struck ten, thanked Deidre for the evening.

"I'm on an early tomorrow, I must go."

She opened the front door, and Deidre, close behind, slipped an arm around her waist.

" You don't want to stay the night?"

Gabrielle turned to face her, shocked.

"Deidre, you have the wrong woman, I'm sorry if I gave you the impression that I'm anything other than a friend. I'm not gay."

"Whoops, forgive me, why are all the good looking women straight?"

"I thought you said you lived with a woman, May, I think you called her?" Deidre moved backward.

"May is my good friend, neither of us are homosexual."

Deidre shrugged. "You're lovely, Gabrielle, you can't blame me for wanting you."

She laughed, and wished Gabrielle good night.

Driving home, Gabrielle wondered why Deidre had mistakenly supposed she was gay. Perhaps she had been too friendly, although not for a moment had she thought Owen was gay.

 Back in her room, Gabrielle relived the evening, and again wondered why she hadn't realised Owen had a romantic interest in her.

Gabrielle remembered being told about lesbians when she was fourteen. In the dining room at school, eating lunch with other students, a male student commented.

 "You can bet Graham hasn't a clue."

"About what."

"Lesbians."

Gabrielle was confused, "A clue about …?"

"Graham, your friend is one."

"Marilyn.? I'm not sure what you mean, and she isn't my best friend, not that it's any of your business."

"Run around with gays, then, who cares?"

"Finish what you're saying, what are you insinuating?"

"Your mate sleeps with women."

Gabrielle was horrified. Sleep with women ? Did he mean have sex with women?

She jumped up from the table, her face burning, and made her way back to the classroom.

Her last lesson was at four pm. after which, she went straight to her room, thinking about Marilyn, who had been in the same primary school as she, when they were younger.

They had bonded, and become friends over several years, although Gabrielle had friends at home, with whom she had a closer tie.

She couldn't imagine Marilyn being sexually interested in her. Although, on several occasions, she had wondered at Marilyn's very affectionate hugs, some might say, 'cuddles', when they hadn't seen each other for a few days.

She shuddered; it was inconceivable that women made love to other women. It wasn't something she had heard of before.

Thinking of her relationship with Marilyn, she remembered receiving a card on Valentines day, which read, 'We were meant to be together.'

It was unsigned, and there was a love heart and kisses at the bottom of the card.

For a while after that, she watched the male students in her group, and in the second and third year groups, wondering if her admirer was one of them.

Since none of the young men paid her the slightest attention to her, she thought it unlikely. That it might be a female never occurred to her.

She had been raised in a home where both parents were professional people and very conventional.

Sex was not a subject that was discussed, although at the private school she attended, she had been taught certain basic anatomy and physiology lessons.

There had never been any mention of women loving women. Did that mean that men could fall in love with men, also. She was appalled at the idea and spent much of the night in tears.

Chapter Twenty Five

In her twenties, gradually, she accepted the idea that same sex relationships were as relevant, as heterosexual pairings. She firmly believed that same gender attraction was not a choice, it was a genetic predisposition.

Why shouldn't same sex partners love each other and raise a family together. She mused that she had come a long way since first hearing of same sex attraction.

She recalling how, after spending the night in disbelief and tears, she eventually came to terms with others' choices, gradually becoming a firm advocate for same sex couples.

She had once been asked by a patient, what she would do, if a child of hers had confessed their attraction to a member of the same sex.

The young man had recently told his parents, he was in a relationship with a boy they thought was his best friend. He had been unceremoniously told to leave, and his parents anger and harsh words had devastated him.

That evening, he had broken off the relationship with his lover, visited a wine store and purchased a bottle of vodka, which he had consumed. He was found unconscious by his flat mate Linda, who called an ambulance, and he was admitted to Accident and Emergency in a critical condition.

After a stormy convalescence, he was admitted to a psychiatric facility where Gabrielle worked, and been directed to her group. Not everyone supported Simon, however Gabrielle permitted no hostility, and those who were offended by same-gender relationships, kept their opinions to themselves.

They were there, Gabrielle reminded them, because they each had something in their lives which had caused them to be sent for psychiatric evaluation, and help.

"Here, we support each other, we do not blame or reject because of our personal beliefs or choices, as long as those beliefs and choices do no harm to others."

Her group were well acquainted with the sentiment.

Answering the young man, Gabrielle said.

"I would be sad, because society is so punitive regarding same sex relationships, having said that, I would support any child of mine in their life choices, emphasizing, that as long as their partner was respectful and supportive of my child, I would welcome them into the family."

She smiled, recalling Simon saying. 'I wish you were my mother,' and the group laughing.

Her last waking thought, was if seeing Owen again on the ward would be awkward for either of them, and that Owen was brave, to put herself in a potentially compromising situation. On the ward, things progressed as usual.

Matron was rarely seen on the ward, and her first ward round with Dr. Crawford was smooth sailing, he was jovial, and obliging. She overlooked the fact that he referred to her as 'Matron,' after telling him several times, that she was Sister Graham, not Matron.

She made certain to look at the medication charts, after he wrote several drugs for different patients, reminding him that it was the eighth, not the seventh, of the month. Smiling, he amended the charts.

After he left, she was in no doubt, that he was suffering from a degree of memory loss, associated with a traumatic brain injury: she would be very careful when working with him, to check everything he wrote on patients medication charts and in their notes.

Where else but in a country hospital would this be necessary?

The following evening, on a late shift, a young girl with an ankle injury came into the hospital, accompanied by her mother. The twelve year old had been playing basketball and landed awkwardly hurting her ankle. Dr Crawford answered the phone call, and within minutes was at the hospital.

Gabrielle had prepared outpatient notes, and Angela was resting on a chair with her foot elevated on a footstool.

Crawford smiled at the child, saying. " Let's taking an Xray of your foot to exclude a fracture."

Gabrielle and Mrs. Robson helped her hobble into the Xray room, and, once the procedure was over, the child was assisted back to the examination couch.

Dr Crawford stood next to Angela, with Gabrielle slightly behind him.

"I need to check that you haven't done any more damage, my hands might be cold."

Angela said nothing, although she seemed unusually flushed.

Gabrielle moved so that she could get a better view of Angela's leg, and to her amazement, she saw that Crawford had his fingers inside the girl's shorts.

Gabrielle elbowed him to one side.

"Dr Crawford, may I see you outside."

She stood aside so that he had no option but to leave the room. She smiled at the girl's mother.

"I just need to check something with Dr .Crawford. "

She wondered if Angela would tell her mother.

Outside she made sure there were no other staff present, leading the way into the office.

"How dare you assault a patient?"

" She's a child, a twelve year old!"

"I have every intention of reporting this to the police."

Crawford shrugged. "I'll deny it."

"The child will uphold my claim."

Crawford said nothing, but left the office, looked at the wet films, and returned to the patient.

" No fracture, Sister will put a supportive bandage on your ankle, stay off it for a few days."

Gabrielle put the bandage on, telling Angela's mother.

"Give her some Panadol if the ankle causes her pain, and if you're at all concerned about anything, whatever that may be, I'm here."

To Angela, she said. "I expect you to tell your mother of anything at all which is troubling you, anything; I'm sure you understand ."

Angela, pale now, and with her lower lip trembling, remained silent, but nodded.

Mrs. Robson asked, " You mean pain, or when she could put weight on it?"

Smiling to reassure Mrs. Robson, Gabrielle replied.

 "I know Angela will tell you if anything is amiss."

"Thank you Sister, I'm sure she'll be all right.

There was no doubt in Gabrielle's mind that the girl would deny the assault if asked.

Gabrielle was incensed.

So Crawford would go unpunished, and no doubt repeat the assaults unless one of his victims in the small town was brave enough to ignore the censure of the townsfolk and file a complaint of sexual assault against Crawford.

Since working at Andover, she had become aware that many of the residents here had never travelled across the border to South Australia, or been further than Nhil, the next town on the Victorian side of the border

Without being critical, Gabrielle thought that many country folk were inclined to be small minded, and that accusing Dr. Crawford would, perhaps, damage the teenagers credibility; particularly since she had not told her mother.

Gabrielle had the impression that this wasn't the first time Crawford had offended. Whether it was as a result of his head injury, she had no idea, furthermore she didn't care.

What troubled her was that apart from May, she had no one to talk to regarding the seriousness of the situation and no idea how to make Crawford stop.

From now on as long as she worked at Andover, she would watch Crawford like a hawk. He would find it impossible to assault another patient whilst she was on duty.

Other people certainly had an impact on the life of innocent bystanders, although Gabrielle would never describe herself thus.

Sister Owen was on a three to eleven shift the following day and greeted Gabrielle with a smile.

"Still fighting the good fight?"

"Not sure I'm winning the battle."

"Need a shoulder? Mine's always available."

Gabrielle laughed. "You really are incorrigible."

Handover was soon finished, Owen asked.

" Anything I can help with? Forgive my saying, you seem distracted."

Gabrielle was silent, wondering if telling Owen was prudent. Owen waited patiently.

"You'll tell me in your own time."

"I'm sorry, just something that happened and I'm still wondering how to deal with it, thanks for the offer."

"Any time, no strings….."
The next day, Gabrielle was in the office when Crawford appeared.

" There you are, I've been looking everywhere for you. Miss Benson wants help to go to the toilet. "

"There are two enrolled nurses on the ward."

"They're busy, you're not."

"I beg your pardon; I don't need someone like you to tell me how to do my job."

"That's too bad, I know you're an Agency R/n, if I let them know I'm not happy that you're caring for my patients as well as I would like, I'm sure they wouldn't be happy."

"Go ahead, I couldn't care less what you do. One more assault on a patient and I won't turn a blind eye."

"Assault, isn't that a bit dramatic?"

He grinned. "I didn't hear her complain, did you? Just in case you forget, her mother was there, she saw nothing, so nothing happened."

"You're disgusting, exploiting a child. You need help. Patients aren't safe with you treating them, you make mistakes, all the registered nurses….."

He stepped closer. "Finish the sentence."

Gabrielle stood her ground.

"You need psychiatric help; you're not fit to be treating patients, get treatment before you do something that'll get you struck off."

"Threatening, are we?"

"If you want to take that as a threat, it's your choice. I care about the patients, I don't give a damn about you, you're a disgrace to the medical profession."

He loomed over her. "Watch what you say, in a court of law you wouldn't have a leg to stand on."

"Be that as it may, I'll be right behind you the minute you walk through the doors."

Shrugging, he turned and walked out of the office, Gabrielle on his heels.

With a grin, he said," Enjoy the rest of the day."

Gabrielle was shaky when she returned to the office, knowing Crawford was malignant enough to make her life difficult.

She could watch Crawford, when she was on duty, she could not monitor him twenty four hours a day, and since emergencies came to the hospital day, and night, he had ample opportunity to abuse a vulnerable patient.

Owen had said that Crawford had been a locum for several years. She wondered if there were people living in Andover who carried the dark secret of being violated by him.

In all her years of nursing she had never encountered a situation like this.

She had been inappropriately touched on a couple of occasions, by a Registrar, and a physiotherapist, and gave them both short shrift.

She was well able to look after herself. A patient subjected to fondling by their doctor, how did they deal with that? Worse, how does a twelve year old make sense of it?

Deeply troubled, she made the trip to Adelaide on her days off, thinking about May's shock on hearing about Crawford, and Gabrielle not reporting what she had witnessed?

She heard Crawford's voice in her head.

'Her mother was there, she saw nothing, so nothing happened.'

The man was a predator, taking advantage of his medical degree to prey on the vulnerable. The thought made her nauseous, worse still, was she complicit in not reporting it?

She was a nursing professional, not a paralegal.

May was welcoming as usual, and after Gabrielle had taken her coat off and sat down, May said. "There are a few letters for you, and I've made cottage pie for dinner, so when you're ready we can bring out trays in here."

Gabrielle was unusually pale, and seemed to have lost weight over the last few months.

"How's work?"

"May, I've never known anything like the kind of things I come up against working in the country."

"It's archaic. I feel so alone."

"At Andover, Matron's never around when she's needed, not that she's much help anyway, but it's her responsibility to keep things running smoothly."

"Things aren't running smoothly?"

"May, I don't think I should burden you with this"

"As the song says, that's what friends are for."

Gabrielle told May about Angela being brought in by her mother and what had followed.

"He wasn't examining her thigh for an injury?"

"His fingers were up inside her shorts, hopefully she was wearing briefs."

"That's appalling, didn't her mother realise what he was doing?"

"No, she was standing behind me so she couldn't see him."

"…and the girl said nothing, she didn't try to move away?"

"May, she had nowhere to go, it's not a wide examination couch, besides which, he's her doctor."

"Jesus, that's unbelievable, he's right, who would believe you?"

May, so proper, blaspheming.

"If her mother saw nothing, the girl made no sound, and you were the only one who saw what he was doing, he's right, it's your word against his."

"Could you talk to Angela.?"

"Not on her own, she's a minor, she'd have to bring her mother or father in, and since she didn't say anything, when it was happening…."

May shook her head.

" That's how predators get away with what they do, their victims are too ashamed or frightened to report the abuse."

"I have no idea how you handle this, even if you tell Rebecca, you've no proof."

"The only way you can stop him is if Angela tells her parents, and you're a witness"

"That's not going to happen, you've no idea how backward some of these townsfolk are, I don't mean to be judgmental but they're pretty close minded."

"In the meantime you're losing weight and having to deal with him, and there's no one to support you. "

"It's been a nightmare. There is one person in whom I could confide."

Chapter Twenty Six

She told May of her dinner with Owen, and despite herself, laughed at the expression on May's face.

'Are you making this up? She thought you were gay?"

"Indeed she did, she was really accepting of being refused. She knows something's wrong, however I wanted to get your opinion before I told anyone else."

"Then tell her, she's there when you're not, she can make sure he's not left alone with a patient"

"Only at the hospital, May, he's got a practice in town."

"One thing at a time , Gabrielle, you'll get overwhelmed if you go at it hell for leather."

Again, despite herself, Gabrielle laughed.

"Hell for leather? May, where do you come up with these expressions? "

Laughing, Gabrielle followed May into the kitchen.

After dinner, they watched 'Pride And Prejudice,' and Gabrielle lost herself in the Bennett's trials, and tribulations. In bed that night, she decided to tell Owen of Crawfords' conduct.

The following two days were spent with May, shopping, dining at one of Adelaide's Chinese restaurants, and relaxing.

Back in Andover the following evening, she phoned Owen, asking if they could meet as soon as Owen could manage, she said she had an afternoon off duty if Owen could make it then. The following morning she had the opportunity to talk to Owen briefly.

"I'm intrigued. Have you decided to bat for the other team?"

Gabrielle laughed. "No, I need some advice."

"I'll see you this afternoon then."

Smiling, Owen left the office.

Gabrielle had to admit Owen was very appealing, and hopefully, she would also be supportive.

The morning passed quietly, and Gabrielle had lunch in the dining room, then went to her room to change into civvies. She had agreed to meet Owen in town at the coffee shop.

Owen was waiting, coffee in front of her.

"Hi, I didn't order for you, I wasn't sure what you'd like."

Gabrielle ordered a latte, then sat down, taking a sip of her coffee.

"So, are you going to keep me in suspense?"

"What I'm going to tell you is sensitive, I must be confident that it stays between you and me."

Owen put her head on one side, looking at Gabrielle intently.

"You need have no concerns about that."

"Thank you, I wasn't sure who I could rely on, certainly not Matron."

"Too true, mate, she's a bloody disaster."

Taken aback, Gabrielle laughed. "I wouldn't have put it quite like that, but I agree."

"You Brits, so correct…"

Gabrielle laughed again.

"I've been told that before."

"So………?"

"I was on duty on Monday evening, when Angela Robson came in with a sprained ankle, I phoned Crawford, and while he was examining her, he sexually assaulted her."

Owen said. " Not the first time that's happened."

"What?"

"Last year, Angela's team mate, Christine, said he'd fondled her, when he was supposed to be examining her."

"She was on her own, her parents were in Nhil, and she didn't say anything at the time, although one of the enrolled nurses told Matron, when Christine came out of the examining room, she was crying."

"They just thought she was in pain."

" So he does what he likes, with nothing to stand in his way?"

"So it would seem."

"When you've been on duty and he's called in, does a nurse accompany him when he's seeing a female patient?"

"What do you think? He says, 'don't worry nurse, I know you're busy."

"That has to change from now on, when you or I are on duty we go with him, he mustn't be left alone with a female patient of any age. "

"The trouble is, he didn't start working here until after he suffered a head injury, so we don't know whether he was abusing patients in Adelaide, although I doubt it."

"Adelaide's not Andover."

"Amen to that." Owen grinned.

"Can the other R ,n's be relied on to accompany Crawford?"

"Only if Matron orders it."

"In that case I'll talk to her."

"You're my hero."

Owen finished her coffee.

"Not sure about that, however I'll let you know how I go."

Gabrielle walked back to the hospital determined to see that Matron agreed to Crawford having a nurse with him when he was with female patients.

She knocked on Matrons' door, and after several minutes the door opened.

"Sister Graham, what can I do for you?"

She made no effort to welcome Gabrielle into the flat.

"Matron, I have to talk to you about something that happened before my days off."

"You'd better come in."

Matrons' dog ran towards her, barking and wagging its tail.

"Benjy, sit."

Matron motioned Gabrielle to an armchair.

"Sister Graham, you couldn't wait until the ward round?"

"No, please forgive me for what I have to tell you."

Matron sat, unspeaking.

Dr. Crawford touched a young female patient inappropriately, on Monday."

"Sister, Dr. Crawford is well respected in the town. Are you sure....."

"I'm neither blind nor a liar. He had his fingers inside Angela Robson's' shorts."

"She complained to you?"

"I saw him do it."

"The girl didn't complain,? Very unusual."

"Matron, Dr. Crawford must be accompanied by a nurse every time he sees a female patient."

"Sister Graham, that isn't your decision to make."

"Then I have no option but to report what I saw to the police."

Gabrielle was aware that the woman was very pale, and there was sheen of perspiration on her face.

Her voice trembling, she asked. "Is that a wise decision ? Dr Crawford....."

Gabrielle interrupted her. "He's either accompanied or I make it public. If Angela had told her mother….."

"Good God, her mother saw it?"

"No, she was behind me, I insist that he isn't allowed to see a female patient without a staff member present."

"What will I tell him? Dr. Connell never needs a nurse with him."

"Dr. Connell isn't a paedophile."

Matron gasped, and leaned back in her chair, tears in her eyes.

Gabrielle waited.

Eventually, Matron said, "Could you fetch my bag, it's in the kitchen, and a glass of water?."

Gabrielle could see the refrigerator in the room opposite, she entered the kitchen, found the bag, and returned to the sitting room.

"My angina tablets……."

Gabrielle shook a tablet into the woman's hand. That explained her failure to administer the hospital, as she should. She had a heart condition.

Gabrielle stood by the chair. "Do you want me to phone Dr. Crawford, Matron?"

"No, no, give me a minute, I'll be alright."

Gabrielle stood, undecided. Matron was pale, and sweaty, was she about to have a myocardial infarction, a heart attack?

After some five minutes, with Gabrielle taking the woman's pulse, Matron's colour was returning, her breathing slowing, and her pulse less erratic and in normal rhythm.

"Will you have a cup of tea.?

"Please, I'm sorry about this."

"Matron, I'm sorry. There just wasn't an easier way to tell you."

Gabrielle found the tea caddy, and laid a tray with two cups, milk, the teapot, sugar, and some biscuits.

Matron was sitting upright now, obviously feeling better. Gabrielle moved a small table next to her and put the tray down.

"Will I pour your tea?"

"Please, milk, no sugar."

"Have a couple of biscuits, they'll raise your blood sugar."

Matron smiled. " I regret we had to become acquainted in this fashion."

"Matron, no more than I. I've been really torn about what to do since Monday."

"My dear, you should never have been put in that situation, It's about time I retired. Ever since I had a heart attack last year, I haven't been able to do my job as it needs to be done. "

"I thought I'd be able to do much the same as before the heart attack. The sad truth is I can't, and it's time to pass the reins to someone who can."

Gabrielle sat quietly, drinking her tea, unable to think of anything to say.

"Someone like you…."

"Matron…."

"Pearl, my name is Pearl, and if you've no objection, I'll call you Gabrielle."

"Please do; may I refill your cup?'

"Thank you, you wouldn't consider applying for the position of Matron?"

"No, I'm not sure how long I'll stay in Australia. With the Agency I can take work on a short term basis. I couldn't do that if I took a permanent job."

 "I suppose not, a pity, Landover needs someone with your integrity."

Gabrielle smiled, "I was really anxious about talking to you, I wasn't certain that you would be supportive."

" Well, now you know why I've been so lax in my job, perhaps you'll understand how difficult it's been to watch what's happening and not be on hand to sort things out. "

"The least disturbance and my heart goes haywire. I should have retired when I became ill, but I didn't have enough to retire on."

"I hope you know that what has happened here is between you and I, there's no reason for anyone else to know."

"I'm indebted to you, Gabrielle. Would you consider acting as my deputy matron whilst you're here, unofficially, of course."

 Thank you, yes, I would like that, we can work together, and you can be assured I'll do my very best."

"Thank you. I think I'll go and have a rest, I've every confidence the hospital is in good hands."

"May I help you to the bedroom?".

"Thank you."

 Gabrielle left the flat scarcely believing what had transpired. Back on duty, she called the two enrolled nurse into the office and told them that in future, any doctor who wanted to see a patient must be accompanied by a member of the nursing staff.

 Both nurses looked surprised,

 Nurse Abbott said. "Dr.Crawford doesn't like a nurse with him."

"Matron wants all doctors to have a nurse present, Dr. Connell and Dr.Crawford will be so advised."

Chapter Twenty Seven

The following day, Dr. Crawford made a ward round, accompanied by Gabrielle. The round over, Crawford walked into the office.

"What's this about a nurse being in attendance when I see my patients?"

"Matron thinks it's appropriate to do so."

"Told the old bird, did you?"

Gabrielle ignored him. He stood contemplating her.

"This round to you."

Receiving no reply, he left the office, Gabrielle accompanying him to the door.

"My, you missed your calling. You should be in the police force."

Watching him walk away, she thought that his gait was unsteady, she knew he often used a walking stick, but she had never realised he was so unsteady on his feet.

A cyclist was brought in, that evening, he had hit a branch in the road and come off his bike.

Gabrielle checked his vital signs, he had been wearing a helmet, so his injuries were superficial, with the exception of a deep laceration on his calf.

Gabrielle gave him a gown, and asked him to take off his clothes. She turned her back, and after several moments, on turning around, realised he was still fully clothed.

"Do you need help ? Your clothes have to be removed so that…"

'Matron, I can't take my clothes off."

"Sister, I'm not Matron. You can't take your clothes off because…….?"

Frowning, he handed her a small glad wrapped package.

"My stash."

"Sorry, your….?"

"My stash, pot, marijuana…. I don't want this getting into the wrong hands."

"It's such a small amount, would that get you into trouble?"

"Better believe it."

"I'll keep it for you."

He was surprised, but made no comment as Dr Crawford entered the room accompanied by an enrolled nurse.

"Thank you, Nurse Abbott, I'll stay with the patient now. "

Crawford examined the young man, and found nothing untoward. Leaving the man to dress, Crawford said. "Sister, I'd like a word with you."

Following him to the office she left the door open. He reached across and pushed it closed,

"I don't appreciate being followed everywhere when I'm in the hospital."

"All doctors will be accompanied by a staff member."

"You're starting to get on my nerves, You're responsible for this; Matron has nothing to do with it."

"Nevertheless…"

He flicked her cheek hard, then pushing past her, he walked to the door, obviously agitated.

She stood, stunned at the outrage. Nurse Abbot came into the office, looking at Gabrielle curiously.

"Sister, excuse me, Mr. Hardy wants to make a phone call."

Gabrielle nodded. " Help him into the foyer."

"Sister, are you all right? Forgive me, you're very pale"

"I'm alright, thank you, Dr. Crawford isn't pleased with having a staff member with him."

Nurse Abbot said nothing, a troubled look on her face.

The staff were aware of Crawford's hostility towards Gabrielle. She went into the staff toilet and looked in the mirror.

She was pale, apart from a reddened area where Crawford had flicked her cheek. She was astounded that he was prepared to use his anger against her in such a physical way, and in a public place.

It gave an indication of the turmoil his brain was in, and boded ill for future meetings with him. She did not doubt that he was in need of urgent psychiatric support. Returning to the ward, she joined the enrolled nurses assisting in bed making and other activities of daily living.

The early shift was trouble free, Crawford wasn't needed, and Gabrielle went off duty, looking forward to meeting up with Owen. In the coffee shop, Owen sat brooding, her face lighting up when Gabrielle joined her.

"I thought you were standing me up."

"Sorry, I needed to pick up a script from the chemist."

"Crawford didn't come in?"

"Thankfully, no."

Owen asked Gabrielle how she was finding Matron's order of medical staff being accompanied by a nurse.

Gabrielle was silent for a moment, then replied.

" Difficult. Crawford is angry about it. Still, he isn't psychologically stable; he shouldn't be treating patients."

"Only the Medical board can prevent him from practicing, are you prepared to go down that path?"

"It might come to that."

She told Owen of Crawford's conduct that morning.

"What a bastard. You're right, he's not stable. That said, you can't accuse him without having substantial evidence."

"Deidre, I've been making copies of medical notes, patients medication charts, and anything Crawford has been involved with. I told Matron of his assault on Angela Robson; she was sick about it."

" Matron hasn't been around much since she was ill last year."

"What happened?"

"She was in Sydney, attending a conference. All we heard was that she'd been taken ill, nothing about what the illness was. She was away for a couple of months, and she was very different when she came back."

"How was she different?"

"She was always around before; she insisted that the R/n on duty kept in touch with her about anything out of the ordinary, even at night; the hospital was her pride and joy."

" When she came back from sick leave, she'd lost weight, and she spent most of her time in her flat. The R/n's pretty much ran the place themselves. You can imagine how successful that was."

"Trouble?"

"We aren't trained as administrators. Between Matron being unavailable, Connell unreliable, and Crawford mad as a cut snake, it was bloody purgatory."

"What kind of things happened?"

'Medication mistakes, the sister in charge had to check anything Crawford prescribed, he would write a medication on the wrong patient's medication chart, or, the correct chart, but the incorrect drug."

"We got in to the habit of only calling Crawford for emergencies we couldn't handle ourselves. Dicey, but there was no alternative. When he was here, we watched him like hawks. All the nurses knew he was untrustworthy."

"Untrustworthy, that's putting it mildly; he's entirely unhampered by scruples.."

"Well, the things that happen here would never be tolerated in a city hospital, although doctors protect each other. We've all heard horror stories of patients being injured, or even dying because of a doctor's mistake."

"Sadly, yes, I worked in a hospital in the U.K. where a patient had an amputation of the wrong leg."

"What happened?"

"He was diabetic, he went to theatre, and neither ward nor theatre staff marked which leg was to be operated on, so the wrong leg was amputated. He sued and was awarded a massive payout".

" He wasn't able to have prosthetic limbs, because of his unstable diabetes and the risk of infection in the stumps, so he was wheelchair bound."

Owen whistled, "Damn, that's rough."

"You're not wrong, Still, when you think of doctors working twenty hour shifts, then going off duty on call, and having to survive on four or five hours of interrupted sleep, it's no wonder mistakes are made."

"Does it make you want to give up nursing?"

"I think it's even more important to continue. If nurses didn't look after a patient's welfare, who else would?"

"Still, you've had a rough time since you've been here."

"I've come to the conclusion that because I trained in a big London hospital, I'm seen as a threat."

"Much as I'd like to disagree, I think you're right. I've heard one or two negative comments. Jealousy, no doubt, your nursing practice can't be faulted."

"Thank you Deidre, I have to admit, I've doubted myself since coming to Andover. If it weren't for May, and you, I think I would have gone back to England, with my tail between my legs."

"Mate, that…I'd like to see."

They laughed, and Owen said. "You're not alone, give me a shout if it all gets too much."

"Likewise, although I don't think you need a hand in standing up for yourself, I can't see anyone taking you on."

"I had four brothers, I was the only girl; they were protective, but they didn't mind giving me a hard time. I learned at a very early age not to put up with bullshit. In case you haven't picked up on it, I swear like a trooper as well."

Gabrielle laughed. "No…really?"

Owen's face was solemn. "I wish you were bi…"

"As Mick Jagger said, 'you can't always have what you want."

Owen laughed. " As if he knew anything about not getting what he wanted, he's a right raver."

Gabrielle returned to the hospital feeling a sense of relief, Owen was courageous and an ally, she wasn't intimidated by Woods or Crawford.

Furthermore, she too, would make certain Crawford did not see a patient on his own.

She invited Owen to dine at the local restaurant the following week, which Owen gladly accepted, both knowing they would remain friends when Gabrielle left Andover.

At the end of the evening, she said goodnight to Owen and walked back to the hospital. Entering the hospital grounds, she heard footsteps behind her, and turning, saw Crawford coming towards her.

" Just the person I was waiting for."

Gabrielle tried to move past him, and he blocked her way.

"Not so fast, I want a word with you."

Gabrielle looked around her, she had her handbag but nothing to defend herself with if Crawford went beyond talking.

"Nothing to say?"

" Kindly get out of my way."

"….and if I don't?"

"I've nothing to say to you."

He seemed unsteady, he took several steps towards her, and she backed away.

"Not so brave now are you?"

"I'm going to report you to the A.M.A. They can deal with you."

"You bitch, don't ………..."

To her horror, he fell forward, and she managed to stop him from striking his head as he fell. She made certain he was on his side, then ran into the hospital. Sister Moffat was in the office and looked up in surprise as Gabrielle came in.

"Dr. Crawford's collapsed outside; can you call an ambulance, then give me a hand?. "

She picked up a sphygmomanometer and stethoscope, and without waiting for a reply, ran outside where Crawford lay unmoving.

She loosened his tie, pulled his arm out of his coat, and took his blood pressure. Two hundred and forty, over one hundred and eighty, she had no doubt that Crawford had suffered a cerebral haemorrhage, a brain bleed.

Moffat had joined her, staring in disbelief at Crawford lying on the floor.

"Could you get a blanket to cover him? "

Moffat disappeared into the hospital.

Gabrielle hoped she had managed to get the ambulance service to send help. There was nothing more she could do to aid Crawford. When Moffat returned, Gabrielle asked if an ambulance had been called.

"They're on the way. What happened?"

"He was leaving as I came in, he just keeled over."

The lights of the ambulance lit up the courtyard, and the two ambulance men jumped out, greeting the two R/n's.

"I'll carry on here, Sister, if you want to go."

Moffat nodded at Gabrielle and left.

The ambulance men looked at her.

" I'm Sister Graham, Dr.Crawford is a locum here. I've taken his blood pressure; it's two forty over one eighty. He has a history of an acquired brain injury."

"Thank you Sister, we'll look after him now."

Gabrielle went into the office.

"Will you phone Mrs. Crawford, or do you want me to"

'Would you mind?'

"Where's the phone book?"

Moffat passed it across and dialed the number. There was no answer.

"Perhaps she's out, will you try later?

"Of course, will he be alright?"

"I doubt it, I think he's had a cerebral haemorrhage."

"Oh no....."

"His B/P was two hundred and forty over one eighty, I've no doubt he's had a brain bleed, malignant hypertension, I would imagine, given his medical history and his erratic behaviour."

"He has been behaving peculiarly, I thought he was having trouble at home."

Chapter Twenty Eight

Gabrielle was torn between wanting to know what had happened to make Crawford so unstable, and not wanting to gossip.

"What makes you think that?"

"I heard his wife shouting at him, he drove off and left her standing in the car park. She was ropeable."

"Well, she won't have to worry about that again, he's on his way to Adelaide."

Gabrielle stood, ready to leave.

"It's too late to wake Matron now, I'll let her know in the morning about Crawford. Dr Connells' back tomorrow, so we'll have medical cover, have a good night."

Although she was tired, she slept poorly, and wondered if Crawford had survive the journey to Adelaide.

There was no doubt in her mind that Crawford's elevated blood pressure had a lot to do with the head injury he suffered previously, and his peculiar behaviour, particularly towards her.

She had a late shift ,and having breakfasted, she knocked on Matron's door, which was slightly open.

"Matron, it's Sister Graham."

Gabrielle pushed the door wide, and Benjie ran towards her, barking.

"Benji, here, good boy.."

She bent to stroke the dog's head.

Advancing further into the flat, she heard Matron call, "Gabrielle, I'm in the bedroom."

Gabrielle followed the dog into the bedroom.

Matron was sitting on the bed. "Good morning, I was on my way in."

"Good morning, I wanted to see you before you came into the hospital, Dr. Crawford collapsed last night and was taken to Adelaide by ambulance, I thought you might prefer to phone the hospital to see how he is."

"Had he been drinking?"

"No, I took his B/p, which was two hundred and forty over one eighty, so it was when, not if, that he would collapse. I couldn't reach Mrs. Crawford so perhaps you would contact her?"

"Gabrielle, she wouldn't be interested, they've been on rocky ground since the accident. She's back in Melbourne with her family, and I don't have a phone number for her, so, status quo."

Gabrielle nodded. "Dr. Connell is back today, so we have medical cover if needed."

"I'll walk over with you, how's everything going?"

"No problems with the patients, I'm on a three to eleven shift, so Sister Moffat will let Dr. Connell everything he needs to know."

At the hospital door, they separated, Matron entering the hospital, and Gabrielle continuing into town, where she stopped at the chemist, catching sight of a delightful teapot, with an owl family hand painted on it.

Remarkably inexpensive, and a welcome addition to her collection.

In England she had a collection of teapots from all the countries she had visited. France, Belgium, Holland, Germany, and two years before that New Zealand.

She had stayed in Wellington for a month, thinking New Zealand one of the most beautiful countries she had ever visited, its weather very similar to England.

Further on, she stopped at the grocers, to replenish her stock of fruit, tea and coffee.

She thought about Matron's remark regarding the Crawfords 'and their marital woes. Further, that the people of Andover could rest assured that their children were safe from predatory behaviour.

Crawfords' collapse had put an end to the probability that she would have to make his behaviour known to Angela's parents, and exacerbate an already intolerable situation.

Rough on him, a life saver for her. Fate certainly worked in mysterious ways. She had seriously considered telling Matron, that she could no longer work in Andover, something she would never have contemplated before coming to Australia.

Connell was certainly unreliable, he wasn't out of control, however.

As long as she had the support of Owen, Moffat, and the other nursing staff, she could manage.

Matron had said she would support Gabrielle's decisions, if medical assistance was unavailable. She knew Matron valued her work, and determined not to be found wanting. Back in her room, she made a cup of coffee, and sat looking out of the window, reminiscing.

When she was a child, she had delighted in the stories told at bed time, by her father, or mother.

The beautiful maiden, rescued by a dashing knight on his steed, was her favourite. Shy, as a teenager, she never had a boyfriend, as all her friends did.

She was twenty when she had her first date, and Matthew, although never a lover, was still a treasured friend.

He had been at the airport, to wish her Bon Voyage, when she left for Australia; she kept in touch by sending him postcards.

Her friends joked, 'Gabrielle will never marry, her knight in shining armour isn't born yet.'

She <u>had</u> found him; he was everything she wanted her partner to be. She doubted she would ever meet any man who had all the qualities Connor possessed.

Until Richard, she had remained a virgin, determined to give herself to her chosen partner only, in marriage, much as her mother, and grandmother, before her. Old fashioned, perhaps, however, she had never considered herself conventional. She marched to the beat of her own drum. Difficult sometimes, not to follow the crowd; to choose her own path, nonetheless, it was who she was.

She knew close friends thought her fiercely independent.

Indeed, she found the notion of being 'incomplete', until she met her 'significant other',

(another ridiculous term), might apply to others, it did not apply to her. She was a fully functioning, intelligent woman, quite capable of being self-reliant, she did not need a man to 'complete' her.

Believing that; she also knew she would marry once only. 'For better, or worse ', certainly her intention. Yet, she had given herself to Richard, the complete opposite of her fairy tale heroes.

That had shaken her confidence in herself, in her ability to make wise, considered decisions. She, believing herself to be foolproof, had moved from England to Australia, to 'marry' a married man, an embezzler, a liar, and a cheat. So much for being independent.

Courageous? Yes. Wise? She laughed, no, not wise. However, she had learned a valuable lesson. Daniel had encapsulated it in his comment, 'what you see, isn't always what you get', or words to that effect. How true. What she got with Richard, was certainly nothing she had expected.

Only her brief relationship with Connor, made her re assess her priorities.

Her passion for Connor frightened her. She had met the man she had dreamed of, since she was a child. Yet, it was never to be. She recalled that as a teenager, her favourite poem was a Shakespeare sonnet, how did it go…?

'Let me not to the marriage of true minds admit impediment, love is not love which alters when it alteration finds, nor bends with the remover to remove…….'

She thought at the time, 'if that doesn't describe true love, I don't know what does.'

A knock on the door, brought her to her feet, and she opened the door to see Owen standing there.

"Busy?"

Gabrielle stood back. "No, come in."

"I thought you'd like to know, Matron phoned the R.A.H. Crawford had a subarachnoid haemorrhage. He went to theatre, and he's back in I.C.U."

"With a blood pressure like that, it was obvious. He was an accident, looking for a place to happen."

"Well, he's gone, we can call off the dog squad."

Gabrielle laughed, " We were the dog squad?"

"Okay, I was the dog squad. In my defence, I would add, I only made the bullets, you were ready to fire them."

Gabrielle laughed again, shaking her head. " Where do you find these expressions, is that 'Strine'?"

Owen shook her head. "No it's not, been looking at Strine, have you?"

'Strine', the way Australians pronounced 'Australian'; which Gabrielle had bought a book about.

Gabrielle remembered being confused, when she had lunched at a café in Sydney, and been asked to pass the' dead horse'. Tomato sauce.

Gradually, she learned that women were 'Sheila's', smoko, a coffee break, sticky beak, a nosy person, Wally, an idiot. The Australians had a slang word for everything, it would seem, and Owen certainly knew most of them.

"Anyway, much as I regret he's ill, it certainly makes our life less stressful."

Talking, they walked to the dining room.

Handover that afternoon was as usual, nothing out of the ordinary to report, Owen said.

Nurse Bankiron was on duty with Gabrielle, and a newly qualified enrolled nurse, Liz Barnes. That evening at six o'clock , Bankiron answered the phone, relaying the message to Gabrielle.

Picking up the phone, she heard male laughter. "Hallo?"

"Oh, yeah, my mate's had too much to drink, he's passed out in the back of the ute."

"Can you bring him to the hospital?"

More laughter. "Yeah, we're jus' down the street."

Bankiron asked Gabrielle if he would be admitted.

"That depends, until they bring him in I can't say. Get a bed ready just in case."

Gabrielle enjoyed working with Bankiron, a motherly, trustworthy ally. She had been to the Bankirons farm when Gwen Bankiron had invited her to dinner.

They were a big, noisy family, typically Australian, Gabrielle surmised.

She had been welcomed, and made a fuss of, Gwen telling her family, 'she's not stuck up, like other Brits we've known.'

They worked well together, and Gabrielle was always glad to know that Bankiron was working with her, when she looked at the roster.

Almost as soon as she put the phone down, the ute drove into the driveway, and Gabrielle went to assess the situation. The three men, wedged into the front of the ute, were in good spirits.

"Which one of you is the patient?"

"He's in the back, Matron"

Gabrielle walked to the back of the ute, stunned to see a deeply unconscious man, lying on his back, convulsing. His mates joined her, no longer laughing.

"You said he'd been drinking? How long's he been like this.?"

"Coupla hours, I reckon."

The speaker, a carrot topped youth , holding a can.

" Can you and your friend take him into the hospital?"

Bankiron was standing at the door, holding it open.

"Might have known it was you lot."

"Hi, Gwen, he's out like a light."

They carried him in, Bankiron directing them to a single room, where they laid him on the bed.

 Gabrielle addressed the red headed youth.

"Wait outside, please, I need some details from you about your friend."

To Bankiron she said. "Take his observations, let me know, and start a chart for him, I'll phone Dr Connell."

"I'll fetch in the oxygen cylinder, keep it on a flow rate of five litres; while I get some Ventolin into the nebulizer; I'll be back with some adrenaline."

Returning to the office, she phoned the Connells home phone number. The call went to voice mail.

"Dr. Connell, a young man 's been brought in, convulsing, and deeply unconscious. His face is swollen, His friends say he's been drinking, but I think something else is going on, can you come to the hospital as soon as you get this message, please.."

Returning to the side ward, she asked Bankiron.

"What's his blood pressure doing?"

"Sister, it's only ninety over seventy."

Gabrielle had a tongue depressor, and asked Bankiron, to hold the man's mouth open, as she expected, his tongue was swollen.

Bankiron said, " he's not an alcoholic, why's his tongue swollen?"

"He's having a severe allergic reaction to something he ate, or drank."

" Take his B/p again, I want to talk with his friends."

Outside, she asked his friend. " Is he allergic to anything, do you know?"

"Bee stings, he's got an EpiPen."

"Has he been stung, possibly?"

"Not sure, we were leavin' the pub, and he rubbed his neck, an' swore."

"Did he say why?"

"No, but by the time we got to the ute, he was really shaky, then he fell over, so we chucked him in the back of the ute. We thought he was pissed, sorry Matron, drunk"

A severe anaphylactic reaction to a bee sting. Gabrielle ran to the office, and unlocked the medication cabinet, located the epinephrine, and a syringe, then ran back past the startled young men, waiting in the foyer.

Bankiron checked the vial of epinephrine, and Gabrielle injected the solution intramuscularly, into the young man's outer mid-thigh. He stirred, but remained unconscious, although his face was less congested.

Gabrielle took his blood pressure, after a few minutes, relieved to see it was one hundred and ten, over ninety. She smiled at Bankiron.

"His B/p is up, we'll continue with the Ventolin, and I'll put in a Jelco, in case he needs an I.v. Could you fetch a tray with the usual stuff?"

Bankiron was back in a minute, and Gabrielle put the Jelco into a vein in his wrist, leaving Bankiron to put a wide Elastoplast over the needle, while she took his blood pressure again.

" Excellent, 140/110, he's no longer in danger of cardiac arrest."

Bankiron said softly. "Good call Sister, Connell not answering his phone as usual? Thank the Lord you were here."

"He carries an EpiPen, so he has a known bee sting allergy, I'm wondering if he'd been drinking, and was too slow to react to a bee sting."

"Bankiron said, "He's a nice lad, keeping the wrong company, this'll make him rethink his priorities."

"He's not out of the woods yet, we'll just monitor him, and pray Dr. Connell gets here soon."

At Gabrielle's request, Bankiron had phoned Philips' parents, as soon as he regained consciousness, and they were by his bedside, both pale, but assured that he was much improved.

By ten o'clock, having had another injection of intramuscular adrenaline, Philip had regained consciousness, and was able to sit up and drink several glasses of water. Gabrielle removed the Jelco. By eleven p.m. when the night staff came on duty, Philip was greatly improved

Sister Moffatt knew Philip, she was a friend of the family, and, after seeing him, she came back into the office, clearly relieved that he was in a satisfactory condition. Gabrielle gave the report on the other patients, then told what had transpired with Philip. His parents knocked on the office door, saying he was asleep. Was it alright to leave him?

When told he would probably be discharged , after Dr. Connells' round in the morning, they thanked Gabrielle, with tears in their eyes.

Moffat, also thanked Gabrielle, who smiled.

"I'm glad I was on duty, although, I'm always around, when I'm not having days off, and I'm always ready to help."

She was well aware, as were the others, that her training in England, had given her skills that the other R/n's didn't have.

She went off duty that night, thankful that her training had been carried out in the finest hospitals in England.

The following day she worked an early shift. She had arranged with the Agency owner, Rebecca, to take a week off, it had been over a year, since she had taken time off.

May was meeting her in Melbourne, and, when Gabrielle went to morning tea break, she joined Owen at the table in the dining room.

Owen knew Melbourne well, telling Gabrielle the best way to get there from Andover, and what to do in the city. With a smile, Owen said.

"Any chance of going along?"

"Sorry, May and I are meeting in Melbourne."

"Worth a shot, you'll be missed."

"Anyway, you travel from Andover, and join the Western Highway, straight to Melbourne, it's very well signposted."

Gabrielle smiled.

" Thanks, I need a break, it's been a long time since I've had time to relax and enjoy Australia."

"I'll take the car in for a service when I get off, and get a few things for the trip."

Owen patted Gabrielle on the shoulder.

"Enjoy Melbourne, half your luck."

Gabrielle was ready early the next morning, and eager to get started. She skipped breakfast, and farewelled Andover, heading towards Nhill. The sun was on the horizon, as she entered Ballarat, heading towards Horsham. As she drove, she pondered on her life since she had arrived in Australia.

Australia was so very different from any of the countries she had visited previously. Certainly, it was nothing like England. She wondered what her parents made of her letters home. She laughed aloud, imagining their faces, when they read her description of the annual cockroach Cup race, held in Karratha, Western Australia.

In each heat, cockroaches, which had been taken from water pipelines nearby, were raced over a twenty two centimetre course. Cockroaches were sold to participants, who viewed them in the specimen cup, with the cost of cockroaches from one hundred and fifty, to over four hundred dollars.

The winner of the race earned its owner one thousand dollars, and cockroaches were named after certain club members. The race, now in its twenty ninth year, was hotly contested, and sixty two cockroaches, six in each race, kept the onlooking crowd cheering, and clapping.

Following time honoured tradition, the cockroach was eaten, after it had won the race In twenty seventeen, one young man whose cockroach won the cup, divided the insect, and shared it with his partner; he was reported as saying, 'it tasted worse than last year's 'roach'.

Chapter Twenty Nine

Involuntarily, Gabrielle shuddered, remembering the newspaper article, about a contestant in Florida, dying after eating over two ounces of mealworms, and part of a bucketful of discoid cockroaches, in an effort to win the prize, a python, owned by the reptile shop,

Gabrielle wondered if the unfortunate man had suffered an anaphylactic shock, since cockroaches were known to store large amounts of uric acid, bacteria, and nitrogenous waste.

Anaphylatic shock. She wondered whether Philip had been discharged from Andover, and would continue to spend time with the friends Owen had called, 'no hopers.'

She was glad that May knew her way around Melbourne, Gabrielle was entering the outskirts of Melbourne, and traffic was congested.

She followed the signs to South Bank, and the Crown Towers hotel, where she was meeting May. She left the car to the valet, and entered the hotel. May was waiting for her in the lobby, and the two hugged, May saying.

"It's so good to see you, let's get your suitcase taken up to the room, and have lunch in the dining room." "We can't check in until two o'clock.. We have a deluxe twin room, so there are two Queen beds, and there's a Wi-Fi, and internet, if you need it."

"That sounds good, also, I didn't stop for breakfast, I ate an apple on the drive, so I'm hungry."

May smiled. "I stayed here a couple of years ago, the food is marvellous, and you can choose which restaurant you'd like to eat in."

They decided to eat in the Conservatory, which had a huge range of international cuisine. They both opted for dishes from the Chef's collaboration, and seated themselves in the huge opulent restaurant.

 The dessert bar was amazing, every conceivable dessert on show. Again, they chose similar dishes, from the Chocolate fountain. Chocolate brownies, fondue, and mixed berry compote

. Brazilian coffee was enjoyed, and replete, they made their way to the via the lift to the fortieth floor where the card unlocked the door to their suite. The views were incredible,

Gabrielle happy that she had bought a camera before she left Andover, as a backup for her trusty Leica S .L. Two.

The room, too, was luxurious, Gabrielle was impressed by the attention to detail shown, for the Crowns' guests. May always stayed at the Crown, when she visited Melbourne, and she was amused at Gabriel's' enthusiasm. They had a list of things to do during their stay, all new to Gabrielle.

They left the room and took the lift to the lobby and reception, where the receptionist phoned a valet to bring the car to the hotel entrance. May asked Gabrielle if there was anything in particular she wanted to do first.

Since it was three thirty in the afternoon, they agreed that visiting the shops in Swanston Street would be enjoyable.

Gabrielle parked the car in one of the underground car parks, and they took the lift up to the first floor, and walked out onto the busy street, which was renowned worldwide as the busiest tram corridor, covering two point eight kilometres.

They browsed in Arthur Daley's, and at Mays' suggestion, walked across to Melbourne Central, where some two hundred and ninety shops were located. May told Gabrielle that it was designed by a Japanese architect, and opened in nineteen ninety one.

It was without a doubt, the biggest shopping area Gabrielle had ever visited, over six storeys high.

Eventually, resisting the temptation to buy any of the tempting items on offer, they found their way back to the car. May wanted to take Gabrielle to Lune Croissanterie, where world class croissants were made, in a temperature controlled glass room, the dough prepared over a three day period.

They joined the queue of people outside the busy shop, and, finally at the counter, choosing two almond croissants, two Pain au Chocolat, and two ham and Gruyere.

May asked Gabrielle if, instead of stopping for lunch when they went to various locations around the city, they could have a croissant.

She directed Gabrielle to the Royal Arcade, where Gog and Magog, the mythical giants, struck the chimes of the arcade's clock every hour.

They wandered around the enormous area, May saying that the arcade was the oldest surviving arcade in Australia, known for its elegance. Gabrielle marvelled at the glass roof, and rows of arched windows to store rooms over the shops.

At the South end of the arcade, they looked at the figure of Father Time, Chronos, which was a feature of the arcade. They had decided to visit the National Gallery the following day when they had more time.

After looking at all the arcade had to offer, they returned to the car, and made for the hotel, in time for a quick shower, and change of clothes, before dinner.

Gabrielle was a keen fan of Japanese cuisine, and May said that the Nobu had a spectacular view from the restaurant. they were escorted to their table, and given the menu. Gabrielle chose the classic yellowtail sashimi with jalapeno, from the menu, and May, black cod with miso.

They marvelled at the one eighty decree views, from the river Yarra, on the South bank, to the docklands, as they enjoyed their food. At last, weary after their long day, they returned to their room, and looked out of the window from their room on the fortieth floor.

The view was magical, the beautiful city lit up, and the picturesque Yarra sparkling. The room, too, was luxurious, and Gabrielle laughed at the deep bath tub, with its built television set. May chose to bathe, and when she had gone to bed, and was reading the hotels' many offerings, Gabrielle took several photos of the city below before pulling down the blind.

They were keen to go to Hosier Lane, to see street art by skilled artists; and the graffiti and political comments which covered the public buildings.

Many tourists thronged the lane, taking photos, and admiring the art. Gabrielle took photos, and commented to May that a lifetime in Melbourne's vibrant city, would never be long enough to experience all on offer. Lastly, they joined a walking tour group, to explore Melbourne's dark side, visiting true crime spots, from bank robberies, to murders.

The slum quarter, Little Lon, was well known for its brothels, and gangsters, where illicit drugs, 'lollies' were easy to procure. Fitzroy , the oldest suburb in the central business district, was said to be the home of criminals, considered by police to be very dangerous, in the early nineteen hundreds.

Speakeasies, 'grog shops,' abounded, and for two hours, May and Gabrielle listened , spellbound, to stories of confectionary shops, used as covers to sell drugs.

Gabrielle knew that the word, 'Speakeasy', also called gin joint, and 'blind pig', came into being, because patrons spoke very quietly, to avoid detection, whilst inside the illegal establishment. By late evening, they were ready to return to the hotel for dinner. They chose to have room service, and Gabrielle phoned to order from the dinner menu.

At quarter to seven, May answered a knock on the day, standing aside to let the immaculately dressed waiter push the trolley into the room, greeting them with. 'Good evening, may I serve your meal ?'

The table, situated in the window, overlooking the city, was laid with a snowy tablecloth, and their selections placed on the table, beside fine china, and shining flatware. Smiling, the waiter bid them enjoy, and left the room. May had chosen Atlantic King Salmon with potato rosti, carrot puree, and broccolini.

Gabrielle inhaled the aroma of the Wild Mushroom Risotto, with sauteed wild mushrooms, and leeks, in crème fraiche. Neither wanted dessert, Gabrielle telling May that she would have to work hard to drop any weight she no doubt gained since staying at the Crown.

As they ate, May, who was always enthralled by Gabrielle recounting various nursing experience, listened, as Gabrielle continued the story of Christmas morning, at Redcliffe, a psychiatric facility in London.

" I worked an early shift, seven to three thirty p.m., and there were twelve patients on the ward, different diagnoses, chronic schizophrenia, paranoid schizophrenia, Bipolar Affective Disorder, and a couple of patients with personality disorders. All the patients who were allowed home leave had left for the day.".

" We had the usual duties, I'd been in on my day off to decorate the ward, and the staff bought small gifts to put under the tree for the patients and staff on duty."

"We had television on and some of the patients sang Christmas songs, along with the singers on t. v. We served breakfast, I gave out medication, and Jenny Crane, who has a guitar, and a really good voice, asked for requests from everyone".

" We served mince pies, and coffee, and it was a really enjoyable morning. The lunch trolley came in, and I couldn't believe it. Turkey roll, mashed potatoes, and carrots. Christmas dinner, it was pathetic".

" The two enrolled nurses, who hadn't worked on Christmas day before, couldn't believe it either. They both commented on how awful the food was. The trolley wasn't heated, and by the time it was brought from the kitchen to the ward, it was cold. We decided to provide Christmas lunch ourselves."

"I phoned my friend, Chloe, remember I told you, May, that she and I were renting a flat together? "

"Anyway, she arrived on the ward, bringing my tablecloth, the turkey, which had been part cooked, the night before, and I put in the oven before I left that morning, along with the ham, and pork, and cauliflower cheese."

"We heated the potatoes in the microwave, and the gravy in the trolley was okay, so, we all sat down to a decent Christmas dinner. The Christmas pudding and custard in the trolley was really good, we pulled crackers, ate, and had a fine old time."

"After dinner, we opened our presents, I really enjoyed that Christmas, best of all, the patients loved it."

"When the late shift came on duty, the patients were happy, and relaxed."

" Chloe and I took the rest of the food she'd brought in, and we still had enough for our guests, the next day."

May smiling, said. "Hospital food is renowned for its inedibility, is that a word?"

" I was surprised when I had a few days at The Grange, the private hospital, in Adelaide, and the food wasn't anything to write home about."

"I ate in the cafeteria."

Gabrielle agreed. " The best hospital food I ever had, was at the Adelaide clinic, really awesome chefs there."

They left the table, taking their coffee with them, to sit in front of the window, and look at the city, lit up by lights from the towering high rise buildings, the tiny cars, on the roads at ground level, and the shimmering Yarra river.

Gabrielle had taken photos of the scene, and couldn't resist taking more. This was their last night in Melbourne, and for Gabrielle, it had been a magical time. Something she could call on when she was stressed and feeling downhearted.

Buffet breakfast at seven the following morning, was sumptuous. The array of dishes was stunning, and Gabrielle walked slowly, looking at the hot and cold dishes. Fresh fruit, pastries, and the usual breakfast dishes, cereals, eggs, cooked in every possible way, bacon, sausages, mushrooms, tomatoes, croissants, and muffins.

Every kind of bread, and a vast array of dairy foods, cheeses, yoghurt, pancakes, blini, was presented. Truly, a gourmets' delight. Neither chose a large breakfast, neither May nor Gabrielle were big eaters.

May had chosen to return to Adelaide on the coach, not wanting to make Gabrielle return to Adelaide, then drive back to Andover. After breakfast, they hugged, and went their separate ways, and by midday, she was back in Andover, the small town seeming very quiet, after the bustle of Melbourne.

She admitted to herself, she wasn't overjoyed about returning to the hospital.

The last few months had been taxing, and she knew, that although Dr. Crawford no longer posed a problem, however the lack of medical support, and Matron's inability to be at the helm of the trained nurses, would mean the final weeks at the hospital would be as stressful as those she had already experienced.

She would tell Matron that she was prepared to work for another fortnight, then she would return to Adelaide. There was no doubt Matron knew how arduous the job was.

 She had confided to Gabrielle, in a moment of weakness, that in the many years she had worked with Dr Connell, she had seen his attendance at the hospital decline, hinting that he had become heavily dependent on alcohol in the last few years, putting patients at risk, and leaving her and the R/n on duty alone, to cope with casualties.

That the stress had contributed to her atrial arrythmia, and subsequent illness, when she was in Sydney, was in no doubt. Gabrielle held her tongue, and Matron apologised saying that she had no one to talk to.

 Regarding the problem of the lack of medical support, she said she had told Dr. Connell of her concerns on several occasions, and he had brushed her off..

 If she reported his conduct and the lack of medical care available to the Medical Board, he would probably be deregistered, therefore, she had no option available , to change the situation.

He had been a friend over the three decades she had worked with him at Andover, indeed , she was godmother to his youngest daughter. Gabrielle felt sympathy for Matron.

Connell's alcoholism, she saw no need to call it anything other than it was, placed his patients in a dire situation. It caused distress among the nursing staff, who undertook medical procedures they were unqualified to perform. Weeks ago, Owen had said that the hospital relied heavily on Agency staff.

'No one with any sense wants to stay here when they realise what a potential disaster it is. Look at what you've had to do since you've been here'.

' Treating Philip for an allergic reaction, supposing you'd been wrong? It doesn't bear thinking of. That's not something you would do in Adelaide.'

Gabrielle didn't disagree. Connell's choices left them all vulnerable, and much as she disliked abandoning a job, she could no longer stay where she was at risk of being deregistered because she had not only made a diagnosis of a patient's condition, but treated the condition without the authority to do so.

Yet, when faced with a situation, similar to the one she had recently encountered with Philip, what other options had she?

To let him deteriorate and more than likely, die? Regardless of the consequences to herself, she would have done exactly as she did. No, difficult though it was, she had no option but to leave Andover.

Chapter Thirty

She longed to return to Adelaide, to May, and the support and comfort she offered. Mostly, she longed for news of Connor. The months away, thinking distance would ease her ache for him, had proved fruitless. If anything, absence had certainly made her heart grow fonder.

The following week was uneventful, and with four days to go before she put Andover behind her, she prepared to go on early duty. At eleven that morning Dr. Connell phoned to say a fourteen month old baby boy was being brought in by his parents, with a burn injury.

Gabrielle could put some Polysporin on the area, and he would see the baby in his clinic on the following morning. The young parents came in, the father carrying a screaming toddler. Gabrielle asked him to bring the child into a room, so that she could look at the burn.

Meanwhile, Bankiron was comforting the sobbing mother. Gabrielle asked the baby's father to hold him, while she gently removed his clothing, meanwhile asking the man how the baby was burned., and learning that he had pulled a saucepan of boiling water over himself.

When the wet vest was removed exposing the small chest, Gabrielle gasped involuntarily. From under his chin to just above the pubic area, the skin had peeled back leaving the flesh beneath visible.

Appalled , Gabrielle asked the father if Dr Connell had seen the baby. The father said that he had been told to bring the baby straight the hospital.

"Did you tell him how bad the scald was?"

"He was impatient, he just repeated that we must bring Jonathon into the hospital."

"Mr. Randall, this is a serious injury, Jonathon will need skin grafts and intravenous fluids, there's a risk of infection. The baby needs to be admitted to the Women and Childrens in Adelaide as an emergency."

"Dr. Connell said you could put some special burn cream on it."

"Mr. Randall, not wishing to frighten you, the baby needs urgent assessment, and critical care in a burns unit. We're not equipped here to deal with burns of this nature. I need your permission to transfer Jonathon to Adelaide.

Mrs. Randall had come into the room and heard Gabrielle's plea.

"Adelaide? No. Dr Connell is our doctor; I want him to look after Jonathon."

"Mrs. Randall, Dr. Connell is away until tomorrow. Jonathon needs urgent medical care. I implore you, for the baby's sake, agree to having him transferred to Adelaide?"
Mrs. Randall shook her head.

"Dr. Connell delivered me, I trust him, We'll wait until tomorrow. "

Mr. Randall shook his head, but said nothing.

With tears in her eyes, Gabrielle went to the nurses station, where Bankiron looked at her, questioningly.

Gabrielle shook her head.

"They won't agree to transfer the baby, they ignored what I said."

"The best I can do is give Jonathon some baby analgesic, will you see what there is in the trolley, suitable for a toddler?"

"Sister, I know them well, do you mind if I have a word with them?"

"Go, I'll look in the trolley."

Gabrielle found paracetamol, took a medicine measure, and the bottle into the room.

Bankiron was still talking, turning to check the paracetamol, and the prescribed amount, then Gabrielle handed it to the mother to give to the baby and left the room.

Bankiron returned to the nurses station.

"The bloody stupid woman, she won't agree. My daughter was in the same class with her, she's thick as a plank and he does everything she says."

Gabrielle shook her head.

'I'm documenting everything, I want you to witness it and I'll give you a copy, their refusal to seek prompt medical care could have serious consequences. "

"The child needs an intravenous started, he's losing plasma from a serious burn wound."

"He'll need skin grafts; every minute is precious and they're refusing to listen to advice."

Bankiron said. "Is it that bad?"

"It is."

"What can we do?"

"Nothing except admit him, try to get him to have as much fluid as possible, give him paracetamol, and pray that Connell gets back early tomorrow."

"Shit.….pardon, Sister, I thought it was parents with their first baby panicking."

"No, they saw the scald, Connell didn't."

"He's a f…ing disaster, I've known him for years, he's gotten worse over the years."

"Do you think he knew how bad it was?"

"Mr. Randall said he tried to tell Connell and he was ignored."

"You can't just send the baby to Adelaide?"

"Not without their permission, See if they'll listen to you, offer them a cup of tea, talk to him, perhaps he can persuade her, otherwise the baby's in strife."

The day passed slowly, and the Randall's remained obdurate about transferring the child. At changeover, Owen listened, alarmed at Gabrielle's report.

"Those bloody cretins, 'I've a damn good mind to tell them a few home truths, inbred bloody …..don't get me started."

"I'm sorry you've seen the worst of Andover, since you've been here."

"What do we do about the baby?"

Gabrielle frowned.

"Nothing we can do, it's their son, their decision."

"I'm sorry to leave you to it, oh, I'm triple documenting everything, had Bankiron sign it, and keep a copy, there's going to be mayhem over this."

Owen nodded. "You're not wrong, I'm doing the same."

"Shall I stay a while? Moral support.?"

"Haven't you had enough? No, you go, I'll see you tomorrow."

Gabrielle went off duty, sadly conflicted. She saw no point in telling Matron, thinking that perhaps it was exactly what she should do. However, what was to be gained by telling a sick woman something she had no control over. That was akin to cruelty. Gabrielle had never been so sorely troubled in all her years of nursing.

To leave the ward, knowing the baby was critically injured, needed intravenous fluids, antibiotics, and intensive care nursing, tore her apart. She was powerless, cursing Connell.

Crawford was bad enough; Connell was even worse. these two men had, with no one to stop them, changed the lives of everyone they came into contact with.. and not necessarily, for the better. In Connell's case, ironically it was his absence which caused the problems, not his presence.

Gabrielle spent the next few hours, fighting the urge to go back to the hospital. It would undermine Owen, who was a very competent practitioner. Whatever happened to the child, was in the lap of the Gods.

So she spent another restless night, rising early in the morning, forgoing breakfast and heading to the ward.

Owen , pale faced, greeted her.

" Thank God you're here, the kid's worse, the f…..g parents won't listen to reason."

Together, they went into the room, where the parents sat by the cot. Gabrielle looked at the lethargic baby lying quietly. Not speaking to the parent, she bit her lip, shook her head, tears in her eyes, then left the room, followed by Owen.

"Will you let me take responsibility for what I'm going to do?"

Owen nodded.

Gabrielle picked up the phone , and dialled a number.

"Hello, my name is Gabrielle Graham, I'm an R/n at Andover hospital, in Andover."

"I admitted a fourteen month old boy yesterday with critical burns. No….. no…. he hasn't been seen by a doctor, please arrange for an urgent retrieval."

" Yes…… How soon? …..No…. Polysporin….. No, we've tried to, he's deteriorated since I last saw him…… ..Yes, of course…ok…I'll tell them."

 Back in the office, she said.

"They're on their way, now for the parents."

Followed by Owen , Gabrielle went back into the room.

" I've arranged for Jonathon to be transferred to Adelaide."

Both parents stared, slack jawed.

"You can't………."

"The nursing staff will no longer accept responsibility for nursing a critically ill child."

Owen, meantime, took off the top clothing, and the dressing, and covered the area with a sterile dressing towel, wrapping the baby in a blanket, and taking him to the nursing station.

Together, she and Gabrielle left the disbelieving parents, to their own devices.

Back in the office, Owen said.

"Bloody hell, I've got to take my hat off to you Brits. I wouldn't have the guts to do what you just did."

"What's the alternative? Watch him die because Connell's an alcoholic bastard?"

Gabrielle, hard pressed, saw no need to hold back on her disgust for Connells behaviour.

"You're not wrong."

Gabrielle said. " Could you let the parents know they can go with Jonathon?"

The parents seemed to have lost the will to fight.

Owen thought they recognized in Gabrielle, a willingness to disregard her own welfare for that of their desperately ill baby.

Mrs. Randall said, "I don't want....."

Mr. Randall interrupted her, asking if it was acceptable for his wife to accompany their son, he would lose his job if he took time off.

"Certainly, she can let you know how Jonathon is doing."

Outside , the ambulance was pulling up in the driveway. Two ambulance personnel, one a doctor, hurried into the office, greeting the R/n's. Owen had removed the blanket and the dressing gently, leaving the sterile towel over the burn area. Both men stared at the baby's chest, disbelief plain on their faces.

Swiftly, the medical team went into the small operating room, and the baby was laid on the operating table.

Scrubbing his hands, Dr. Prior said.

"Cut down, I'm afraid, his veins are too collapsed for an intracath. "

"You said he was admitted yesterday, and not seen by a physician?"

Gabrielle replied.

"The parents were told to bring him to the hospital, he would be seen by the doctor today."

"Was the doctor told the extent of the burn?"

"Evidently."

Gabrielle watched as the impossibly small vein was expertly located, and the intracath inserted. The baby cried weakly, and both nurses watched, with tears in their eyes.

Finally, with the essential intravenous fluid going into Jonathon's system, he was dressed in a gown, wrapped in the blanket, with his tiny arm on the board to keep it stable, and taken into the ambulance.

Gabrielle had never been so relieved to see a patient leave the hospital, even though it was not a discharge.

Owen said.

"Coffee ?"

"I haven't had breakfast yet, too late for the dining room now, and you're off duty."

"Bugger that, this is a day I'll never forget."

"You certainly have a way of changing the script."

Gabrielle laughed.

"Some scripts need changing."

"Bankiron's on, she'll give a shout if she needs a hand. Let's get you fed."

They went into the kitchen, and Owen made coffee, while Gabrielle put bread into the toaster. Owen said.

"Couldn't do this at Q.E.H, or the Royal Adelaide.".

"There wouldn't be a need, Jonathon would be recovering now, not starting on his journey."

"True; it's made me rethink my priorities. I can't stay here any longer, I've had a gutful."

Gabrielle winced.

"Matron will be devastated, she can't get reliable R/n's, Agency staff are not permanent, and no R/n with good qualifications wants to spend too long away from a big hospital."

" I'm really sorry for her."

Owen nodded.

"Tough, no doubt she'll be retiring soon, who's ever heard of a hospital where the doctor's a drunk, and Matrons 'a no show?"

"I always respected her, but lately, between her, Connell, and Crawford, it's a bloody horror show."

Gabrielle choked on her toast, coughed, and took a sip of coffee, before replying.

"I'll miss you. You have a killer sense of humour."

"Mate, I'm off to Adelaide, bugger the cottage, I can't let it tie me down here any longer."

"Seeing you in action's made me realise what a slack unit I am."

Gabrielle laughed.

" Do you mind letting me finish my toast before I choke myself?"

Owen smiled.

"At the risk of boring you, I'll say it again, you're my dream come true. What you did took so much courage"

Gabrielle smiled , and nodded.

"This place has certainly tested my courage. Off to bed, with you, I'll see you later."

Owen nodded.

"In all seriousness, thank you, you're an exceptional nurse."

"Thank you, you're not too bad yourself."

Telling Bankiron she was going to see Matron, Gabrielle went to the flat, and knocked on the door. Benji barked, as the door opened.

"Gabrielle, good morning, I'll be over in a tick."

"Matron, there's something I must tell you, before you go to the hospital."

"Not more trouble?"

"Unfortunately, yes."

She told of what had happened the previous day, finishing.

"He's on his way to Adelaide, his mother with him, and I'll phone before I go of duty, and let you know how he is."

" I can't tell you how sorry I am, that you've had to deal with this, I've made up my mind to resign, and Dr Connell must face the consequences of his actions as best he may. I won't shield him any longer."

"Rest assured, my dear, you have my one hundred per cent support. It took a great deal of courage to do what you did."

"I regret you won't be the hospital's next Matron; however, I appreciate that you belong in Adelaide."

Talking, they walked back to the hospital, where the drama of the previous hours might have been a dream.

Two days later, Gabrielle waved goodbye to the staff assembled outside, to see her off. Matron had hugged her, as had Owen and Bankiron, promising they would stay in touch.

May was waiting, and as Andover became a dot in the background, Gabrielle knew she would miss the three who she had farewelled, as for everything else, it would be a not always welcome memory.

She had phoned Rebecca to tell her she was returning to Adelaide, and while happy to take short term work, would not be available for a country appointment.

To Rebecca's enquiry, she replied. " Best I come in, to let you know how it went." Despite Rebecca's entreaties, she refused to be persuaded. What had happened at Andover would take time to explain, and understand. Gabrielle could hardly make sense of it herself.

Soon, she was entering the Adelaide suburbs, and, it was with a sense of gratitude , that she parked the car, and walked into May's welcoming embrace. She would take at least a week off before she accepted another job.

May had a tray ready, and insisted Gabrielle sat down, while she made coffee.

"There's gingerbread, made this morning. You must have some."

She was concerned to see that Gabrielle had lost even more weight, and was pale, seeming despondent.

"Let me know what you think about the gingerbread, it's made with molasses, which gives it the deep colour, and that heavenly taste."

Gabrielle sipped her coffee, and cut a thin slice from the wedge May had put on her plate.

"May, I can't possibly manage all that, I'll cut it into slices, freeze it, and have it with coffee over the next few days."

Laughing at May's expression, she said. "Waste not, want not, I'm not letting you throw this away."

May smiled.

"You can't imagine how happy I am that you're taking a week off before the next job. I mean to get some flesh on your bones, you look so thin."

"May, Andover was a nightmare, I think Jonathon was the nail in the coffin."

"I phoned the Women's and Childrens, he's still in intensive care, he's had the first graft, and he's tolerating antibiotics, intravenously, Sister Giles said, if he's rehydrated by this evening, they'll stop the intravenous fluids"

"They know some of the story, from Dr. Prior, I couldn't say anything else."

"I'm just so thankful that I'm back home, I can leave medical decisions to the medical staff."

"I made a firm promise to myself, I'll never work in another country hospital again."

May nodded. "I'm glad to hear that; I've missed you. You're back where you belong."

So Gabrielle spent the following days recovering from the months spent at Andover. May was a comfort, there wasn't anything Gabrielle felt she should hold back on.

Chapter Thirty One

May had encouraged her to talk about her doubts in making decisions rightfully the doctors domain. Gabrielle's fear that her actions in transferring the baby without parental consent could result in her disqualification. Further, treating Philip with drugs not prescribed by a doctor. All highly unusual, and putting her at risk

May insisted that any intelligent R/n would have followed the same path. They were trained to help patients, not stand by, when the patient was in dire straits.

"Let's hope, the Victorian Nurses Registration Board sees it that way."

"Victorian?"

"May, I was in Victoria, if I'm struck off there, will I still retain my South Australian registration?"

"If it comes to that, how does it affect my English R/n status, if I'm deregistered here in Australia? "

" Don't think I wasn't aware of the mess I might get into. Still, I'd do it again."

"How could you not? Shameful that you and the other nursing staff were put in that situation. "

"Country hospitals, I dread to think what happens in most of them. Owen told me stories that made my hair curl. She stuck it, because of the cottage, after Jonathon, she told me , that was it."

 She's leaving the cottage for the local real estate people to manage. She said it was worth paying them to be rid of the constant anxiety, and fear, that a patient would die."

It's a ridiculous state of affairs, I can't help wondering why the townspeople don't lobby their local M.P."

May stood up, "I'm going to make a pot of tea, then, I'll teach you how to crochet. We can talk, and work."

Gabrielle was a fast learner, before the hour was out, she could manage the crochet hook, and make chains. After two hours, she had made several squares of different colours, and learned how to join the squares, to make a small cushion cover.

May, meanwhile, had finished the shawl, and was looking at knitted toy patterns.

"My grandchildren have quilts, all different colours, and patterns, and toys I made when they were babies. Now I knit or crochet for charity."

Gabrielle had seen, and admired May's work, the artistry was amazing.

 May said. "I was asked by the library to have an exhibition of my work. That was in November, last year. I thought I would be able to do the display myself. I knew how the toys, crocheted rugs, and cushion covers would be best displayed. I left the work there, and when I went in to the library, the display was already completed."

"I could hardly see the display, there was a big crowd, mostly mothers, with their children, in front of the display cabinet. Anyway, at the end of November, I phoned, and asked a librarian, when I could collect the work. She asked if I would leave it there over the Christmas period , it was so popular."

"So, I knitted Santa, and Mrs. Claus, and a snowman, wearing a scarf, and beanie, Mrs. Claus holding a cracker, and Santa, with a sack of tiny toys, a teddy bear, rabbit, and crackers.

They were so tiny, I had to use three ply baby wool, and the smallest knitting needles I could find."

" The display was supposed to be dismantled after three weeks, in November. It was still on display in March. Every time another display was scheduled, the library members objected, eventually, I said I wanted the toys returned. "

" I kept forgetting to take a photo of the work, in the glass fronted cabinet, and just after I asked for everything back, I went in, and there was another display. I really regretted not taking a photo. "

"I was getting phone calls, from people who wanted something knitted to give as a present."

"I got snowed under, I sat for eight, nine hours a day, making toys, until I developed repetitive strain injury , it was so hard on my hands I stopped taking orders, now , I knit for charity."

"May, I don't think I'll ever be as proficient as you."

"Gabrielle, it's like anything else undertaken, the more time, and effort, put in to whatever, the better the result. You're only just learning, and already you've not only mastered the technique, you've crocheted enough squares to make a cushion cover."

"You can use any wool here, I think you'll find it easier to work with a three millimetre hook, and eight ply wool. The guiding rule is, the larger the hook, or knitting needle, the thicker ply, the wool."

When you feel confident, choose a project, and your wool, and, you're all set."

"May, how did I manage, before I met you?"

Gabrielle laughed at May's expression.

By Sunday evening, Gabrielle had learned to knit, and had chosen a pattern for a bear in green shorts, with a green and yellow hat, and a green striped waistcoat.

 In her next relaxation class, perhaps she would tell the group that craft work was not only productive, it was an effective way of easing stress.

Even better, thanks to May, she could demonstrate how to knit and crochet. She had been told by May, that men were some of the best knitters in the world; in fact, sailors were noted for their incredible skill.

On Monday morning, she caught up with Rebecca, who had been concerned about Gabrielle's experience at Andover. She assured Gabrielle that none of her Agency staff would be sent to Andover, until she was assured that it was a safe environment for both them, and their patients.

Gabrielle had opted to work on a day basis, and, since she was qualified to work in a general setting, in a psychiatric facility, or a maternity ward, there was no shortage of situations available.

Her first job was at the forensic services hospital in the northern suburbs of Adelaide. The huge facility was administered by the Correctional Services, accommodating patients convicted of a criminal offence,

They were deemed unfit to plead, because of mental impairment at the time they committed the offence. Gabrielle was fascinated with forensic sciences, and arrived at the building promptly at six forty five.

She entered the reception area, where her personal details and photograph were taken by a correctional officer, then the door was opened remotely. After a series of doors were opened for her, she arrived at the ward where she would work for the day.

This was a first for her, no keys, to open and lock doors. She was welcomed to the ward, and given a report about the three patients she would be responsible for, that day.

There was one psychiatric registered nurse, male or female, for three patients, and Agency staff were expected to read each patients notes. There was no haste, these patients were all capable of caring for their own personal needs.

Gabrielle sat in the office, and selected her first patient's notes. She had two males, and one female patient. When she left the office, she knew that each of the individuals assigned to her for the day, were incarcerated because they had committed a murder.

The woman had murdered her boyfriend, in Darwin. Both she and her partner were Aborigines, with several infant children, who were now in care.

Her first male patient had 'King' hit a passing stranger, who fell, fracturing his skull on the kerb, and never regaining consciousness, dying in hospital a week later, despite valiant efforts by the staff. He was in his early twenties, and had been married only two months previously.

Her third patient had a long criminal history, and was well known to the police.

His M.O, Modus Operandi; (mode of operating) was to 'break and enter.'

An opportunist, he would check the house for a car parked in the driveway. If there wasn't a car, he knocked on the front door, and getting no response, went to the back of the house, broke in, and stole any valuables he found.

On this afternoon, he went through the ritual, and broke into the house, finding a women in the kitchen. He raped, and strangled her. Appalled, Gabrielle read, that the dead woman was a nursing sister, on night duty, who was preparing the evening meal for her family.

The morning passed quietly, with the exception of a small fire being lit in a waste paper basket, by a patient who was incarcerated because he was an arsonist. He was in possession of a lighter. Gabrielle wondered how an arsonist managed to secrete a lighter, since patients were checked for weapons, regularly.

That afternoon, she was asked by her patients to fetch the playing cards, so they could sit out in the yard, and play card games. Sitting in the sunshine, it occurred to Gabrielle that she was sitting at a table, on a sunny afternoon, playing cards with three murderers. She wondered at her life.

Learning to crochet, and knit, and her friendship with May. In complete contrast, sitting and playing cards with patients who had killed another human being. Yet, she was at peace with the diversity of her life.

At three thirty, she had reported on her three patients, checked that she had signed for all medications given, farewelled her patients, and repeated the process of being allowed through all the doors, then signing herself out, and leaving the building.

She had found the day interesting, however, she preferred being able to work in different nursing environments. She thought that working in a correctional service facility was acceptable for a short time, however, she would find it tedious over a prolonged period.

The work offered no challenge, it was strictly controlled, regimented, even. She was glad to return home, May was out, and Gabrielle showered, and changed into a track suit, sitting in front of television, and picking up her knitting. May had persuaded her to start knitting a square. Gabrielle browsed through the dozens of toy kitting patterns, choosing to knit the bear, then decided that, yes, perhaps she should listen to May, start simply, and leave the bear until she was more experienced.

The following day, she worked at a private facility, for patients with substance abuse issues. She was surprised to see a woman she had nursed with at the R.A.H, and greeted her, thinking how nice it was to work with a friend. Then it occurred to her that Emilia wasn't in uniform.

"Hi, you on duty, too?"

Emilia shook her head. "Unfortunately, no, my husband, Warren, is a patient here."

Gabrielle, was silent, unable to think of how to respond.

"It's alright, Gabrielle, I'm used to it. He's an alcoholic, I've lived with the fallout for years. he's just been diagnosed with cirrhosis."

"Em, I'm so sorry, that's awful."

" I've had enough, if he doesn't quit drinking now he knows that's it. I'll keep the house and the kids, he can do what he wants, I'm finished with it."

"Em, do you have some support, your family, a friend?"

"I'm lucky, my family and Warren's are supportive, they're as fed up with him, as am I."

"You didn't read about the latest alcohol fueled caper in the Telegraph, or see it on t.v.?"

Gabrielle shook her head.

"He crashed the car into a drive through in Stansbury, spent the night in the police lockup. Meanwhile, I was phoning his family, friends, various casualty departments."

"We were sick with worry. Of course he wrecked the Mercedes, his pride and joy. I picked him up the next morning, and he couldn't remember anything about the accident....complete void."

Gabrielle had heard the report on the news, she realised, and remembered May's comment.

"Drunk, and driving, what gets into these people?"

She had met Warren several years previously, when Emilia, who liked to be called 'Em,' invited her to a barbeque at their beautiful home.

She had wondered about his air of distraction, and Emilia checking on him constantly. It was very apparent something was wrong. Gabrielle wondered if Emilia wanted to confide in her, hence the invitation to lunch. However the next couple of hours passed, and Gabrielle left, none the wiser. Now she understood what her friend had been struggling with.

An alcoholic husband, whose alcohol abuse resulted in cirrhosis of the liver, and blackouts. He was mid-thirties, so Gabrielle knew he had a good chance of recovery, if he stopped abusing alcohol.

"I'm leaving, you know where I live, let's catch up, I'm not working at the moment, and my parents are looking after Valerie, and Bronte. Call me when you have time off, we'll catch up ."

Gabrielle hugged . "I will, take care of yourself."

Emilia nodded, tears in her eyes.

Nothing about the work was a challenge, Gabrielle very used to interacting with patients with substance abuse issues. Caring for a friend's husband, someone she had met in a social setting, however, presented a problem.

She went to the D.O.N.'s office, and told Mr. Merrick that she knew Warren Parker, and she would not be able to work with him.

"Not a problem, he's off to the Q.E.H, so transport is taking him at nine, you won't see him. Thank you for letting me know. It would have been awkward for both of you."

The day went quickly, and on her way home, she reflected on the people she had shared the day with. She always pondered on the same thing when she nursed patients with addictions.

The difficulty, not only for them, but for their family, because of the substance abuse lifestyle. It was a lifestyle, confronting though it was, for those with an addictive personality. The classical music programme was interrupted by a news flash. She listened as the newscaster said.

'We have breaking news from Port Arthur. Thirty five people have been gunned down, and many more injured, police units, and ambulances are on the scene, and the gunman has been taken into police custody. We will have updates, as more news comes to hand'.

Chapter Thirty Two

Gabrielle pulled the car over into a safe spot, and sat, trying to make sense of what she had heard. She was shocked, and disbelieving. Tears ran unchecked, and she kept the box of tissues on her lap.

She must have been mistaken, surely that had been five people? She sat quietly, until she felt able to continue driving. May was sitting in front of television when Gabrielle entered the house.

"May, is that about Port Arthur?"

May nodded, pale faced.

Gabrielle sat down, looking at the chaos in the Broad Arrow café, and the surrounding area in the historic tourist precinct of South Tasmania. She hadn't been wrong.

Thirty five people, including a baby and several young children had died in the shocking onslaught at the one-time penal colony. Twenty two others treated for injuries, and shock.

Both women sat, silently, numb at the news. Thankfully, the gunman had been detained. Thirty five innocent tourists. Adults, children. It was incomprehensible. For the rest of the day, television was turned off, and May and Gabrielle sat, not speaking for long periods.

Mass killings were unheard of, yet, in beautiful Tasmania, it had happened.

They went to bed that night, without eating an evening meal. May had insisted that Gabrielle had a small glass of whisky. May had several.

The following morning, both were tired, understandably. Fortunately, Gabrielle was not rostered on duty. May and she had a breakfast of toast and coffee, then sat in the lounge, listening to classical music.

Neither wanted to hear any more news about the Port Arthur massacre, knowing that it was one of Australia's darkest days.

They listened to the beautiful Hauser rendition of 'Adagio For Strings.', as they worked on their knitting. Gabrielle was eager to start knitting the bear, and May went through the pattern with her, explaining the terms, and telling Gabrielle, that all the abbreviations were found at the beginning of the pattern, as was the wool ply, and size of the needles.

She was slow, but meticulous, and after several hours, she had knitted the bear's body. They stopped for lunch, then continued with their work. By that evening, Gabrielle had knitted the bear's arms, and both legs. They put the work away, and , unusually May hugged Gabrielle, as they wished each other a good night. Gabrielle was ready and away before May was up, the next morning.

She was on duty at the Q.E.H., remembering her first time there, with the image of Connor bright in her mind. She was rostered to Outpatients, and found it absorbing. It was a huge are, with rooms all around the central seating area. Consultants for every imaginable disease saw their patients in the small rooms, and it was a fast pace.

Throughout the day, Gabrielle heard snatches of gossip, all centred on the Port Arthur massacre. The gunman, Martin Bryant, was unknown to police. He evidently suffered from Aspergers syndrome, and had a history of disruptive behaviour. He was intellectually challenged. An irritable, dim, bullying individual, uneducated, and insistent on leaving school before the age of sixteen. He was befriended by a wealthy woman, who died in a car accident, and she bequeathed her fortune to him. He soon found his wealth attracted neither girlfriends, nor friends in general, rather, he attracted those willing to exploit him.

It was known by police that Bryant had gone into a department store, two weeks before the massacre, and purchased a sports bag, large enough to conceal numerous semi-automatic shotguns.

Try as she might, not to listen, it was all people could talk about, so outrageous was it. Bryant was, evidently, a good-looking young man, with long blonde hair, and blue eyes. Gabrielle thought that Bryant's infamous behaviour had been accepted by those he met in the course of a day, because of his good looks.

In Bryant's case, handsomeness hid his dark personality. In the following months, Prime Minister John Howard banned all firearms owned by those without a permit:

Bryant was convicted in the Supreme Court, and sentenced to life behind bars, in Risdon prison. The Broad Arrow café was deserted, never again the sound of children laughing, of tourists talking, to be heard.

So another day passed, and wearily, Gabrielle returned home.

She welcomed the security of home, and the ordinary pursuits, she was keen to continue knitting the bear, and talking with May, about how she had spent the day.

May was cheered by Gabrielle's return.

The massacre had affected her deeply, as it had many, not just in Australia, but all those who heard the news, around the world.

Everyone who came into contact with Bryant, after the massacre, would live with it, for the rest of their lives.

The police, who arrested him, the medical personnel, who cared for the victims, the lawyers, defence, and prosecution, who worked with him.

Indeed, the families of all those who had direct contact with the smirking, arrogant, notoriety seeking, mass murderer

Bryant's defence lawyer embezzled five hundred thousand dollars from his law firm, buying artwork, and other collectibles, and ultimately, being convicted, sentenced to four years in prison and disbarred from practicing law. Indeed, Bryant claimed many victims. The three patients she had worked with, at the Correctional facility had each killed one unfortunate person. Bryant had murdered thirty five.

May told Gabrielle , she had spent the day in the Botanic Gardens, enjoying the sunshine, able to escape her thoughts for a while.

May, rock steady, reliable, May, reeling at the tragedy.

Gabrielle knew that not talking openly, and avoiding the subject of Bryant, and the horror he had unleashed, was no longer an option.

"May, let me help you in dealing with the massacre, I'm concerned about your mental welfare. Talk to me."

Gabrielle had opened the floodgates. She held May, as her friend sobbed, and spoke in a breaking voice, about the victims, and her grief. Gradually, the flood of tears ceased, and May went to the bathroom, to bathe her swollen eyes.

Gabrielle busied herself in the kitchen, laying a tray with mugs, the teapot, and milk, and the remains of a chocolate cake she had bought the previous day, hoping to tempt May, whose usually robust appetite had deserted her.

May came back into the lounge. " I won't apologise, I know you understand. I needed to grieve; I just didn't know how. I was frightened of giving way to my emotions."

She sat down, while Gabrielle poured tea, and cut a wedge of chocolate cake.

"Try this, it's from Drakes, how does it compare with your chocolate cake?"

May laughed," You're joking, I can't compare what I make with the cakes from there."

Gabrielle smiled. "Don't be modest, you make a bloody good cake."

May, unused to hearing Gabrielle swear, laughed again.

"I give in. When we've had this, we can get on with our knitting. I looked at what you've done, apart from a few mistakes, it's very good. "

"Will you show me how to pick up a dropped stitch? I sorted out a small crochet hook, and next time we go shopping, I'll buy a knitting bag."

"No need for that, come, I'll show you what's up in the loft."

Together, they went up to the loft, and May switched on the light, illuminating the large room.

"Here, this packing case; whatever you need, you'll find here."

Gradually, they brought out items that had been stored for several years. Crocheted rugs, patterns, bundles of knitting needles, small cases with complete sets of crochet hooks, and at the bottom of the pile, wrapped in tissue paper, knitting bags.

"I made these at night school, I even bought a sewing machine, but after the course, I went back to knitting and crochet. "

With a mischievous smile on her face, she asked, "Are you interested in having sewing lessons, if so, the machine's yours."

Gabrielle laughed. "I'll learn how to knit first, then we'll see."

She chose a knitting bag, and they went back to the lounge.

Gabrielle sat quietly, listening to the needles clicking. May had lost the tense look on her face, and Gabrielle knew that although there would be moments of sadness, they would not feel the overwhelming grief they had both suffered.

"I'm taking two months off, after my next job."

May looked up, surprised.

"Two months, what do you have in mind?"

May, will you come to Western Australia with me?"

"That's a long time. Gabrielle, let me think about it, why do you want to take so much time off?"

"May, I'm going home after I've been to Queensland, and Western Australia."

May rose, and knelt by Gabrielle.

" I know you haven't been happy for months; it isn't work, is it?"

"No, Andover wasn't always a great experience, however, I wouldn't let that put me off."

"Connor."

Gabrielle nodded.

"May, I can't work anywhere I might see him, knowing he's out of my life forever. I think about him constantly."

"He makes every other man I come into contact with, work related, or whatever, seem

diminished by comparison; "

May put her arm around Gabrielle's shoulders.

"Do what you need to do, I'm happy to go with you, my family are always telling me to travel."

Rebecca knew that Gabrielle did not want to work at the Q.E.H. for personal reasons, however there was work aplenty anywhere else the experienced R/n chose.

Both psychiatric hospitals in the Adelaide suburbs were being closed down, and Gabrielle agreed to work wherever she was needed. The following morning, she was awakened by her phone ringing. She looked at the time, five forty five. Who would be phoning her this early in the morning ?

As she listened, she turned on her bedside lamp, it was still dark outside.

"Yes I will……around thirty minutes….no worries. Okay, I'll speak to you later, Rebecca."

No time to shower, she washed her face, and dressed quickly, hoping the phone call hadn't awakened May.

Thankfully at this hour there was little traffic on the road, and she made her way to the clinic in record time, identifying herself at reception, and being directed to room twenty four.

She entered the room, surprised to see an R/n she recognized from nursing administration, at one of the psychiatric hospitals being closed down. It was obvious she had been crying.

"Graham, thank God it's you. I've made a right fool of myself."

Gabrielle noted Sister Daniel's pallor.

"What happened?"

"This is my first shift with the Agency, I came on last night, to look after Mrs. Bennett, she was admitted yesterday after a suicide attempt."

"This morning around six, she said she wanted to go to the toilet, so I made the bed while she was in the bathroom. After a while, I knocked on the door, and realised she'd locked it."

"I called to her to open the door, but she didn't answer."

"Then I heard a crash, and I panicked. I raced to admin, and got a spare key for the bathroom door."

"Graham, she tried to hang herself from the shower curtain"

That explained Daniel's pallor and her swollen eyes.

Gabrielle had looked at the unconscious woman, flashed the torch in her eyes to look at her pupils, and taken her pulse, whilst Daniel's was speaking.

Gabrielle said. "Sit down before you fall down, I'll get you a cup of coffee. What's her name, did you say?"

"Laura Bennett, her husband's a sheep farmer in Lucindale. She caught him in bed with their babysitter."

"That'll do it."

Daniel's laughed, her face losing its pallor.

Gabrielle smiled.

"I won't be a minute."

She found the kitchen , and made a jug of coffee, laying a tray with biscuits, and two mugs.

Back in the room, she put the tray on the table, and poured two mugs, pushing the plate of biscuits towards Daniel's.

" Didn't the Agency tell you who you'd be caring for?"

"No, they said it was a female patient, on her way in."

"Dropped you in the deep end, charming, you would have been better working with clinic staff until you had more experience with Agency nursing."

"You know where I'm working's being closed?"

"Another mistake, people in need of psychiatric care being put out into the community, and left to fend for themselves, pretty much. A shameful state of affairs. Too bad politicians aren't made to work in a psych facility for a day."

"Yes, it'll cause chaos. I thought I would try Agency work, I've only got a psychiatric registration, so there's not much option."

"Who's this lady's doctor?"

Doctor Wakefield, he came in this morning, and gave her some I .v .Diazepam, she's been out ever since."

"Good, anyway, she can't be nursed in the clinic, I'll phone him, she needs to be nursed in a secure environment. The clinic isn't it."

"I didn't think so when I read her notes, but because this a private clinic, I didn't know what to do. If only I hadn't let her lock the door."

"Don't blame yourself, the Agency shouldn't have put you in this situation, given it's your first job. When you've written the report, go home."

"I've done that. Will you check it for me?"

An administrator in a large psychiatric hospital asking Gabrielle to check her report. The irony did not escape her. This was a woman used to command, to having others do her bidding. Miracles would never cease.

" Nothing wrong with your report, just put' Agency,' after your signature, then the clinic staff know where to go, if they need to contact you."

"Oh no…do you think they will?"

Gabrielle wrote her phone number on the clinic notepad.

" Don't worry about it. You shouldn't have been put in this situation. If you need someone to talk to, this is my phone number.

"Thanks, I hope Mrs. Bennett's okay, and thank you again, I was about ready to hang myself, too."

They both laughed, and Daniel's left. Mrs. Bennett slept soundly, so Gabrielle decided to look through the suitcase in the wardrobe. Whoever had packed the suitcase, probably the erring husband, had obviously been in a hurry.

There were several diaphanous nightgowns, but only one slipper, and no dressing gown. Two John Grisham novels, a teddy bear, and a bag containing makeup. A large toilet bag., an Aran cardigan , several blouses, leisure wear, and a small case, probably with jewelry inside.

Gabrielle shook out each garment, feeling for lumps in the sleeves, and anywhere else capsules could be secreted; then laying them on the chair. The makeup bag contained several small pill bottles. Gabrielle shook them out onto the table.

Diazepam. Gabrielle had given patients the drug on so many occasions, she recognized it, immediately. She found the key to the case, in the pocket of the leisure wear trousers.

Opening the case, she saw different colored capsules, and pills; most of which she recognized. She counted sixty capsules, all from different manufacturers, and all tranquillizers.

No doubt, Mrs. Bennett had been 'doctor shopping,' either that, or she knew someone in the trade. It was an enormous amount of potentially lethal drugs.

Gabrielle was appalled that a suicidal patients' suitcase had not been searched, initially, by clinic staff.

Patients did commit suicide in hospital settings. She knew of several, who had died by their own hand, traumatizing hospital staff.

Chapter Thirty Three

It wouldn't happen on her watch, she felt compassion for Daniel's, thinking it was more good luck than judgement that Mrs. Bennett had not secreted enough capsules to kill herself with, when she locked herself in the bathroom. She rang the bell and a staff member answered her call.

"Please stay with my patient while I go to the nursing station."

The R/n looked surprised, but nodded, and sat on the chair by the bedside. Gabrielle took the drugs with her, and asked the R/n's in the nursing station who was the senior R/n.

"I am….Sister Dyer, you're Mrs. Bennett's special, I believe?"

"Sister Graham, I want to leave these with you."

Unceremoniously, she dumped the drugs on the desk. Both R/n's looked at the drugs, frowning.

" I would like a signature for them, please , so I can put that into my report."

"These were in her case?"

"Yes, I've gone through everything that came in with her, there are no more drugs. I 'll phone her doctor, and request her transfer to Hall Crest, she's still asleep at the moment, so I'll let her family know, after Dr Wakefield has been in."

Neither nurse said anything. Gabrielle left the office, and returned to the room, thanking the R/n, and asking if she could .arrange for a staff member to stay with the patient when meal breaks were due.

Danielle went to the dining room at midday for lunch. Whatever the nursing staff were remiss in , she couldn't fault the chefs. The food was sublime. Of course, the clinic catered for wealthy, and , on occasion, celebrity patients, so the food would have to be good.

On her return to the ward, Gabrielle sat by the sleeping patient, and waited for Dr. Wakefield to arrive. He was prompt. Tall, professional, and immaculately dressed, he listened to her, interrupting once.

"These drugs were in her suitcase?"

He agreed that as soon as Mrs. Bennett was awake, she must be transferred. Before he left, he asked her name, and thanked her for her care of his patient. Gabrielle wrote her notes carefully, taking a photocopy. At four p.m., Mrs. Bennett stirred, and Gabrielle introduced herself, asking Mrs. Bennett what she would like to eat and drink.

The suitcase had been repacked, and she would be told of the transfer, when she had eaten. One thing at a time. Mrs. Bennett was hungry, and made short work of her food.

" I must go to the bathroom"

"Certainly, may I help you, or are you happy to go alone?"

"I'm fine, I don't need any help."

She went into the bathroom, and Gabrielle stood outside, holding the door open.

"Close the door."

"I'm sorry , Mrs. Bennett, the door stays open."

"Close the f….. door."

"I regret it, but the door stays open."

"Who are you? I'll let my doctor know about this."

"Do, in the meantime, I have a duty of care, the door stays open."

So Mrs. Bennett performed her ablutions under the gaze of her determined R/n, and returned to her bed.

There was a knock on the door, and an R/n quietly informed Gabrielle that the ambulance was here for the patient.

"Mrs. Bennett, Dr. Wakefield wants you to be transferred to Hall Crest".

Mrs. Bennett was outraged. "What? You bitch, you'll regret you were ever born."

" Where's my phone? I won't go.."

Gabrielle stood aside, while the ambulancemen pushed the gurney beside the bed, and asked Mrs. Bennett if she needed help to move across onto the gurney.

"I'm not going anywhere. I'm….."

"If you don't get on to the gurney, we'll have to help you, one way or another, you're being transferred."

Mrs. Bennett gave a wail, but climbed onto the gurney, shouting abuse. Gabrielle followed behind, with the suitcase.

In the back of the ambulance, Mrs. Bennett called Gabrielle every vile name she could lay her tongue to. Gabrielle quietly said that Dr Wakefield had arranged the transfer, for Mrs. Bennett's safety.

"You won't be remembered in her will."

The ambulance man grinned at her.

"What did you do?"

Gabrielle whispered.

"Stopped her from killing herself."

He pulled a face, and shook his head. Mrs. Bennett continued her verbal abuse until they reached the ward, and was put into a room.

Gabrielle gave her handover, and left the suitcase with the nursing staff, who had waited until the patient was in her room, then gathered round to see why Gabrielle had been screamed at.

Gabrielle phoned Rebecca, and gave a brief description of the day's events. Rebecca knew that Gabrielle had worked her last shift with the Agency.

She had been dismayed, that the Agency Daniel's worked for, had sent an inexperienced R/n, to a job where she had no support. She was sorry to lose Gabrielle, reiterating that

Gabrielle was always assured of a welcome, she ever wish to return.

Gabrielle slept soundly that night, Since deciding to leave Australia, she had felt her stress decreasing. She regretted leaving May, whom she treasured; however, she acknowledged that working anywhere she might see Connor was no longer possible.

May had coffee brewing, and the enticing aroma of sausages and bacon scented the air.

"Slept well?"

Gabrielle smiled. "Did I what."

May laughed. "Your parents won't know you; you sound like an Aussie. Breakfast is ready."

Seated, May asked what Gabrielle had planned for the day.

"I have no idea, what are you doing?"

"I was hoping you'd like to go shopping?"

"Why not, anything in particular?"

"I want to take you to the Arcade, and see what the women's department in Myers has on offer. My going away present."

Gabrielle blinked back tears.

"May, great idea, I can get you a going away present too."

May laughed. " Not sure that's how it works, but it's a lovely thought."

Leaving the breakfast dishes, they prepared for the outing, and were soon on their way. The mall was crowded.

 Gabrielle heard the familiar sounds of Pachelbel, played on the violin, by a talented musician. Many artists, studying at the universities, attracted crowds in the mall. Magicians, jugglers, acrobats, all could be seen at various times.

Myers was busy. They took the lift to the women's department, and wandered through the displays. May came over to Gabrielle, carrying a blue dress.

"What do you think of this?."

"It's gorgeous, is it a size ten?"

"Sadly, no, twelve."

Together, they looked for a smaller size, then Gabrielle held the dress against her, looking in the mirror.

"What do you think?"

"It's perfect, will you have it?"

"May, of course. thank you."

The dress paid for, and bagged, they went up to the restaurant for coffee. Gabrielle said.

"After this, let's look for your present."

Downstairs, they wandered through the various departments.

"Perfume, May, would you like perfume?"

After teasing their senses with various perfumes, May held up a tester bottle.

"This is beautiful, This one."

At the counter, the saleswoman smiled.

May blinked at the price.

"Gabrielle, that's too expensive."

Gabrielle shook her head. "May, you'll never use it without thinking of me."

They made their way back to underground parking, and were soon on their way home, both pleased with their gifts. In her bedroom, Gabrielle tried on the dress, which fitted perfectly. She realised she had lost weight over the past few months.

"Gabrielle, you look stunning, the blue is the same colour as your eyes."

"I thought that, too. I'm not sure when I'll get the opportunity to wear it though. Perhaps we can go into Adelaide for dinner one evening?"

"Shall we choose somewhere, and see if we have to make a reservation?"

That done, they tackled the housework, then, in what was becoming a pleasurable habit, took up their knitting. Gabrielle had made the bear, and was knitting the waistcoat.

She had learned how to pick up a dropped stitch, using a crochet hook, picking up a loop in the previous row, directly underneath the dropped stitch, and hooking it up and over to the row on her needle.

While they worked, they talked. May encouraged Gabrielle to tell her about patients she had cared for, and was fascinated with the correctional psychiatric facility.

"You were telling me about the man who killed the nursing sister. What happened to him, do you know?"

" A year later, I was working at the psych: hospital, when we had an admission.

"When both the psychiatric hospitals were closed, leaving only the psycho gerontic wards open, patients were either out in the community, in general hospitals, or sent home. It was a nightmare."

"Anyway, it turns out, the admission was the man I was telling you about. He'd been transferred from the correctional services facility, to the locked ward I was working on."

"I couldn't believe it, this dangerous psychopath, in a locked ward, when he should have stayed where he was. The nursing staff were outraged."

"Mad, or bad?, they said."

May shook her head,

"May, you haven't heard the worst. Six months later, I was in the Mall , and who should come walking

towards me?"

"No. He was out?"

"He was out. This murderous, conniving, devious bastard, sorry, out in the community."

"The Government wanting to save money, closing all the mental hospitals, with only six or seven beds in general hospitals, not secure, and most of the time, the nurses were general, not psych: trained."

"God knows who makes these appalling decisions."

"This young woman, with small children, murdered , and he's out there, living his life."

"You can bet I put my name on the petition, to have him jailed"

May said.

"Let's go out to lunch, we haven't had Chinese for a while, wear your new dress."

They were soon at their favourite restaurant, enjoying their meal, talking, and laughing. Gabrielle said.

"If I keep eating like that, I'll wish I'd picked the size twelve dress,"

Neither had anything else they wanted to do, and were soon back in the comfort of the lounge room.

Gabrielle showed May the sleeve of the bear's cardigan.

"What do you think, is it.............."

They were both startled by the doorbell ringing.

"I'll get it, you stay there."

Gabrielle opened the door.

"Gabrielle, hello."

She stared, disbelieving.

"Connor, what...I..."

"May I come in?"

She stood aside, holding on to the door frame, shaky, feeling her skin blanch.

He put his arm around her.

"Come and sit down, I'm so sorry, I didn't mean to frighten you."

May was not in the lounge.

Gabrielle sat, while Connor went into the kitchen, returning with a glass of water .It was obvious this was not the first time he had been in the house.

"That's better, you're not so pale."

"So you know May?"

"I do, she came to the Q.E.H. and told me you were going home and why."

"How embarrassing. I don't know what to say, I'm sorry."

"For what, loving me as I love you?"

She raised her head, tears in her eyes.

"I saw you, Connor, months ago, with a young woman......"

"May told me. My love, she's my niece Ashley, she's years younger than me, I'm no baby snatcher."

Humour, to lighten the mood. Gabrielle gave a shaky laugh

"Your niece?"

He laughed. "My niece."

He took her hands, and pulled her up and into his arms, smoothing her hair from her brow.

She was aware that he, too, had lost weight. Looking down, he laughed.

"You've been sitting on a bear…"

She laughed.

"May taught me how to knit. I'll let her know you're here"
"Not yet."

He lifted her chin and kissed her. Holding her close, he said.

" I think May knows."

"I can't let you go back to England. You belong here with me. I won't let you go again."

There was a knock on the sitting room door, and May came in, beaming, and carrying a tray.

"Hello, Connor."

"May."

"Who wants a cup of tea?"

Gabrielle burst into laughter.

"May and her tea."

"May, we're celebrating. I can't believe you talked me into buying a dress, and wearing it out to lunch, so that I didn't look a wreck when Connor arrived."

May laughed. "Guilty. I took a chance that Connor cared for you as much as you cared for him."

"Oh May, I've been such a fool, all those months, working around Australia, miserable, and out of my depth."

Connor smiled at May. "May's been busy, she helped me shop, as well. What do you think of this."

Gabrielle opened the small box, and looked down at the ring.

"Marry me, May wants to be your Maid of Honour."

Gabrielle's last thought, before she was hugged by May, and kissed by her fiancé, was, that at last, she had come home.

www.ingramcontent.com/pod-product-compliance
Lightning Source LLC
Chambersburg PA
CBHW022049210326
41519CB00054B/284